1990

The Creative Practitioner

Creative Theory and Method for the Helping Services

ABOUT THE AUTHOR

Bernard Gelfand, MA, MSW, is Professor, School of Social Work, Faculty of Community Services at the Ryerson Polytechnical Institute in Toronto, Canada. He is presently working on a Doctorate in Education, Applied Psychology. He has been teaching individual, group and family treatment methods for fifteen years and for the past nine years has been teaching a course that links creativity and problem-solving methods for the purposes of helping students think more creatively about practice problems and to develop new procedures, programs and policies for the helping services. Professor Gelfand has published numerous professional articles and has also conducted a host of creative problem-solving workshops for human service professionals, teachers, photographers, artists and lay person.

The Creative Practitioner
Creative Theory and Method for the Helping Services

Bernard Gelfand

The Haworth Press
New York • London

The Creative Practitioner: Creative Theory and Method for the Helping Services, is Volume #2 in the Haworth Series in Social Work Practice.

The Haworth Press, Inc., 12 West 32 Street, New York, NY 10001
EUROSPAN/Haworth, 3 Henrietta Street, London WC2E 8LU England

LIBRARY OF CONGRESS
Library of Congress Cataloging-in-Publication Data

Gelfand, Bernard.
    The creative practitioner : creative theory and method for the helping services / Bernard Gelfand.
        p. cm. — (Haworth series on social work practice, ISSN 0898-0705 ; v. 2)
        Bibliography: p.
        Includes index.
        ISBN 0-86656-649-X ISBN-86656-659-7 (pbk.)
        1. Human services — Methodology. 2. Problem solving. 3. Human services — Decision making. I. Title. II. Series.
HV31.G37 1988
361.3′2 — dc 19   87-33795
                                                                    CIP

DEDICATION

To my wife, Dorothy, a truly creative practitioner

CONTENTS

Preface

My interest in seriously studying problem solving started over ten years ago. I began to give undergraduate students assignments that required them to design something new for the social work profession. Surprisingly, I found that some students were quite good at inventing. Other students struggled with these assignments and became immobilized by the thought that they must develop some idea for the profession that supposedly hadn't been considered before. I noticed that the students who enjoyed these "invention" projects approached them in ways that were significantly different from the students who found them so difficult. My initial theory of what made a student inventive went something like this: The students who showed inventive talent were open as persons, were less conventional than others, were interested in a problem that needed a solution, were unafraid to explore the problem and were able to wait until a number of ideas came to them before fixing on one of them. Good, I told myself, these students are *problem solvers*.

So I began to scour the problem-solving literature and discovered that my search of it led me to the domain of creative education. I found that the literature in creative education was rich in theory and technique and this material could be used to help students become better problem solvers. In 1979 I discovered that the Creative Education Foundation in Buffalo offered Creative Problem Solving Institutes each year and I began to attend them, thereby increasing my experiential understanding of how to go about problem solving creatively. My thinking and doing became more sophisticated, and, as it did, I presumptuously offered a course in Creative Problem Solving in the School of Social Work at Ryerson Polytechnical Institute in Toronto in 1980. It was an undergraduate course and the purpose of it was to help students learn to become self-directed as thinkers, learners and doers.

Through the years that I have taught this course I struggled to find reading material that could bridge the gap between the fund of knowledge reposited in the creative education domain and the problem-solving material produced within the helping services. What was required was a text that professed to understand the two domains and to synthesize them. This is the text that I have attempted—one that joins the theory and practice of problem solving with the theory and practice of creativity—for the purpose of identifying a *creative problem solving practice* for the helping professions.

The Creative Practitioner is a text that is designed for undergraduate and graduate helping service students (social work, rehabilitation, corrections, clinical psychology, vocational guidance, etc.).[1] The text is also valuable to helping service educators, who, through its use, can enrich their students' problem solving experience and skill. The third population that the text can serve are those practitioners already employed in helping service positions. Here I am talking about social workers, psychologists, rehabilitation and correctional counsellors and others who serve in a direct service capacity, as a supervisor to others in direct practice or in a higher level administrative position.

How can the text benefit helping service students? Undergraduate helping service students come to their task as helpers with many preconceptions about the helping process. Any helping service educator can recognize the pattern whereby students try to solve a problem before clearly defining it and then produce but one idea for solving the ill-defined mess. The application of the Creative Problem Solving model I espouse teaches students to postpone the solution of a problem until it is defined. Further, students, by learning how to employ the Creative Problem Solving model and its guidelines, become better able to think fluently and flexibly. Because the model requires students to defer judgment they learn to produce many and different alternatives for defining, solving and implementing problem solutions.

The Creative Problem Solving model explicated in the text has

---

[1]Although the text has been tested by social work students the author has offered Creative Problem Solving workshops that have been attended by a variety of helping service professionals and with good results.

value for graduate helping service students too. Those students oriented to direct practice will find the techniques for acquiring the skills of problem definition and generation of alternatives invaluable for inventive practice. Reframing becomes so much easier as a practice skill when the student develops the ability to view a person, problem or situation in a number of ways. Students pointing toward administration in the social services can benefit from an understanding and use of the total model. The model is an invaluable tool for use in program design and development. Its application teaches the value of a strong search of data prior to problem definition, as well as planning in a clear, specific and concrete manner.

Helping service educators will find the text useful in a variety of ways. First, the text can be used to *reinforce* the understanding of the problem solving process in direct practice. Because the text offers exercises in *all* the skills of problem solving the helping service educator can present the problem solving process and its stages, show how the stages are worked through by the presentation of case material and then offer students the opportunity to acquire the skills necessary for helping clients solve their problems. Assignments can be designed by the instructor to augment those provided in the text. For example, once students have learned the technique of producing many problem statements the instructor can provide students with sets of data and ask them to produce a prescribed number of problem statements from the data. Or the instructor may take the process one step further and ask students to converge on the most preferred problem statement and produce many possible ideas for problem solution. Teaching students to expect that there are many ways to solve a problem encourages students to approach their clients with a positive attitude.

The text can be used for a number of different courses. I use it as my major reading assignment for a course labeled Creative Problem Solving. It is offered to undergraduate social workers and I ask that the students taking it creatively approach a problem of their choosing in practice, program development or social policy and to work it through to the planning stage by the end of the course. I have found that by offering them the Creative Problem Solving model and theory and techniques that are linked to it that *all* students can readily face the difficulty of this assignment. Students have developed such inventions as a game to educate and sensitize children about sexual abuse; a kit that combats burnout in child welfare workers; and a multi-media presentation for promoting and advertising services available to the aged population.

The text can also be used as a supplement to a direct practice course that takes a problem solving focus. *The Creative Practitioner* fits well with any helping service approach (model) that emphasizes that practice situations predictably move through various stages, beginning with an attempt to understand what the client system[2] is presenting and ends when the client system grapples with the feelings that attend the ending of formal help.

Finally, the text can benefit students taking courses in administration of the helping services, and, as well, community development. Because the Creative Problem Solving model is so clear in demonstrating how to define problems, produce ideas, decide upon the most preferred solutions, plan for their implementation and to evaluate their impact, the instructor can introduce any part or all of the model for use in program innovation, social planning and organizing local groups for collective action. Students and practitioners acting as locality developers must know and transmit a model of problem solving to groups they are enabling. The Creating Problem Solving model provides a framework that can be taught to students and practitioners, who can then model its use in the locality group.

The Creative Practitioner is *not* being presented as a panacea for all the difficulties that presently beset the helping services. Creative Problem Solving is but one tool that can be found useful by students, educators and practitioners. My belief is that helping service practice can be infused with greater creativity than is now employed. If this book encourages greater efforts in this regard its merits will be assured.

---

[2]Client system, here, refers to individuals, couples, families and groups.

Chapter 1

Integrating Creativity
and Problem Solving

A large number of helping service practitioners and students consider themselves problem solvers. They are socialized within their professional education to view the work of their professional lives as problem solving. As a helping service educator I believe that problem solving is an appropriate goal regardless of the helper's theoretical stance. And I believe this as well: that problem solving, a model of helping that involves certain ways of thinking, must be infused with creativity.

PROBLEM SOLVING – A DEFINITION

Problem solving is a systematic, step-by-step thinking *and* acting process that involves moving from an undesired to a desired state. Problem solving, as a process, begins when I face a disturbing or difficult situation. For example, as a helping service educator I might realize that I am not teaching my practice class as well as I could. My students are not learning. Therefore, I am faced with a difficult situation. How can I solve it? If I am a poor problem solver I will impulsively act overtly to change the situation. But the good problem solver inhibits this action; maintains an open and receptive stance and is willing to entertain a number of suggestions for solving the problem. Rather than changing from a lecture-discussion format to that of straight lecture for my class, I begin to consider other ideas. I realize that a two-hour lecture would be exceedingly tedious and boring for both myself and the students. The class is made up of twenty-two students. Thinking of the conditions of the difficulty (a relatively small class) has made me reject my first solution.

I begin to think in earnest. My class is made up of students who have had some actual helping service experience and some students that have had none. The experienced students participate more in class than the inexperienced. There is little interchange between these two class groups. Rejecting my first idea to solve my disturbing situation has forced me to examine some of the conditions of this situation. And, as I do so I begin to form an idea in my mind of what the problem might be. The situation, experienced initially as upset and annoyance that my class is not learning is being transformed into a *problem*. The felt difficulty has become a *mental* phenomenon. I begin to view the difficulty as a problem composed of the way I am teaching a class comprised of students with different levels of experience.

The solution(s) that now come to me are controlled or guided by the way I have *defined* the problem. A solution to the problem occurs to me. I must encourage cooperation and sharing between the two groups in my class. The experienced students can help the inexperienced students understand field practice through their *actual* experiences. The inexperienced but more conceptually advanced students can help the experienced students view their experiences through the window of theory. This solution, actually a *hyphothesis*, is tried. I form small groups made up of several students from each of the experienced and inexperienced sub-groups. I encourage small group discussion in these groups. Then I form the total class for the purpose of helping all students connect the practical experience with theoretical concepts. In doing so, I am not convinced, however, that my idea is right; rather, I take a tentative stance toward the idea. It is an hypothesis and if it does not work I am willing to reject it. If the class participates and cooperates together, *then*, certain conditions should be found. They should learn the material, as exemplified by better test scores. The students should practice with more confidence and understanding in field placement. I should be able to observe students making connections between field phenomena and theory. By so reasoning, I set up a *test* of my hypothesis. If it works, i.e., if the phenomena I have just enumerated are found, the problem has been eliminated or significantly reduced.

PHASES IN PROBLEM SOLVING

As can be seen in this example, solving a problem involves a series of steps, or phases.

John Dewey, the philosopher and progressive educator, identified in his book *How We Think* (1933), five phases in solving problems. In the first phase we confront a difficulty, inhibit an overt action to overcome it and find a suggestion to solve it. Dewey called this stage *suggestion*. As we correlate the suggestion with the difficulty that confronts us, we enter the second phase of problem solving, *intellectualization*. It is in this phase, as we begin to see whether our suggestion fits the conditions of the difficulty, that we attempt problem definition. The definition of the problem leads us to the third phase that of the *guiding idea*. This idea is further elaborated in a fourth phase *reasoning*, and in the fifth phase is *tested by action*. Figure 1 translates Dewey's phases into the modern day terms used by D'Zurilla and Goldfried (1971), in their exhaustive review of problem-solving theory and research.

CREATIVITY—A DEFINITION

Creativity is a special form of problem-solving thinking. We have seen that problem solving involves a number of different thinking activities—it is a phase-related activity that can occur whenever we are faced with a difficulty we wish to resolve. Creativity is necessary whenever we come against an unusual or unique situation. We must think creatively when we confront a novel situation. For example, it was not difficult for me to think of an idea for attempting to solve my teaching dilemma. But consider a situation for which there are no known methods for solving the problem, say, for example, the design of a space capsule (Adams, 1974). Although we can search our memory for possible solutions we can retrieve none. Ideas, in this case, must be constructed through other thinking procedures than those used in normal problem solving.

One of the earliest definitions of creativity is that by Wallas, who

Dewey's Phases		D'Zurilla and Goldfried
suggestion	←→	orientation
intellectualization	←→	problem definition and formulation
the guiding idea	←→	generating alternatives
reasoning	←→	decision making
testing the idea by action	←→	verification a. implementation b. evaluation

FIGURE 1. A translation of Dewey's phases of problem solving into those developed through a review of problem-solving theory and research.

in *The Art of Thought* (1926) suggested four stages for its execution. An invention or a new idea is brought about when the mind is *prepared* by a deep investigation of the problem. Secondly, comes the stage of *incubation*, an interval of no conscious thought on the particular problem. It is during this stage that unconscious events may work upon the problem to provide fresh ideas for it. Wallas called such a fresh idea or flash of insight, *illumination*. *Verification*, the last stage in the creative process, is worked out consciously and is an attempt to demonstrate the worth of the idea through test.

Consider another definition of creativity, this one put forward by Donald W. MacKinnon, an eminent researcher in the creativity domain. MacKinnon views creativity as a process characterized by a novel response to a problem, in which this response or idea solves a problem or accomplishes a goal, and, lastly, can be evaluated through its achievement in reality(1978, p. 54). (See Figure 2.)

Both Wallas and MacKinnon's definitions of the creative process show themselves to be but variations of the problem-solving process. The creative process differs in respect to problem solving in demanding a novel response or sudden insight to a problem; beyond this difference the processes appear remarkably similar. In fact, what we could say is that creativity and problem solving as processes *merge* under two conditions (1) when the problem faced by the problem solver demands a novel idea and (2) when the problem solver is able to provide such a response. Under such conditions problem solving is transformed into *creative problem solving*.

A PROCESS EXTENDED IN TIME AND CHARACTERIZED BY:

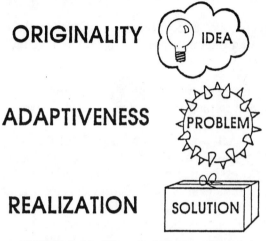

ORIGINALITY

ADAPTIVENESS

REALIZATION

FIGURE 2. MacKinnon's definition of creativity.

Whether we are considering problem solving or creative problem solving is determined by *external requirements*, i.e., the problem presented, and by the creative *capacity* of the individual as problem solver.

THE DEMAND OF THE HELPING PROFESSIONS

Social Work

Does the work of social work require a creative problem-solving approach? In other words, do the problems that social workers face require creativity—novel and unique ideas?

Yes, they do. It is a cliché to say that most human problems are highly complex, almost impossible to sort out as to causality, and frequently resistant to change efforts.

It is not peculiar then that the helping professions, almost unanimously, have adopted a problem-solving stance to the problems it daily confronts. Perlman, perhaps the first major social work author to advocate a problem-solving approach for social casework indicated that:

> the problem-solving model stands firmly upon the recognition that life is an ongoing, problem-encountering, problem-solving process. (1970, p. 139)

Along the lines of a creative problem-solving process Perlman indicated the need in the sequence for a *search* for solutions to the problem (1970, p. 136).

Many other social work authors have allied themselves with a problem-solving approach. Bloom has called problem solving a "design for professional action" and following and expanding upon the general organization of D'Zurilla and Goldfried (1971) has identified a seven stage model of problem solving for social work practice (1975). Bloom is clear about social work's need for creative problem solving; he views creativity as productive rule breaking, a route to better solutions for solving problems (1975, p. 166).

Reid, one of the developers of the task-centered social work system, essentially a problem-solving process, unequivocally views the worker and client roles in finding solutions as a creative activity. In discussing the planning stage of the task-centered system Reid mentions the importance of worker-client collaboration in generating alternatives for problem solution.

> The process works best if both the practitioner and client can freely suggest alternatives as they come to mind, without too much consideration initially as to their appropriateness. (1978, p. 142)

Such a suggestion comes near to the creative skill of deferred judgment as elaborated by Osborn (1963).

Moving away from the realm of clinical practice we can cite Rothman's social R&D model, basically a problem-solving process, as one requiring creativity. The conversion and design stage, in which social science findings must be translated and transformed into prescription and program for practice, is viewed by Rothman as an art requiring imagination and inventiveness different from that used in accumulating knowledge (1980, p. 97). Within Thomas' Developmental Research and Utilization model, which also follows a problem-solving format, is indicated the need for a *generation process*, whereby basic information is transformed through novel assembly, application or invention into product design for new social work procedures (1978, pp. 112-113). I have indicated the importance of creative problem-solving methods for use in the development of new social work inventions (Gelfand, 1982c). In this paper a connection is made between a model of social work research (Thomas, 1978) and creative methods coming from a specific approach to creative problem solving (Parnes, 1977).

Finally, Hepworth and Larsen have suggested a problem-solving model and method for enabling clients to enhance their problem-solving abilities (1983). Their approach advocates the use of brainstorming, a small group method for finding creative ideas (1982, pp. 335-336).

Summary

Although I have not included above an exhaustive review of the social work authors that advocate a problem-solving approach to social work, one that includes either an interest or some attempt to promote a *creative* problem solving, there appears to be a consensus toward a problem-solving stance for social work practice. Other authors such as Compton and Galaway (1984), Johnson (1983), Strean (1978), and Schwartz and Goldiamond (1975) have presented social work practice approaches that either clearly specify a problem-solving approach or one that closely parallels it.

PROBLEM SOLVING
AND OTHER HELPING PROFESSIONS

Social work is not the only helping profession that has embraced a problem-solving focus to practice. Psychology has developed a strong interest in it as an approach to helping people.

Psychologists have long had an interest in problem solving and have studied animals and humans in their attempts to understand this process. D'Zurilla and Goldfried reviewed well over one hundred references to problem solving, both theory and research, in an attempt to relate this work to behavior modification practice (1971). They defined problem solving as a behavioral process which makes available a diverse number of responses for dealing with a problem situation and improves the likelihood of selecting the most effective response from the number generated (D'Zurilla & Goldfried, pp. 107-108). What must interest us in their powerful attempt at synthesizing this literature is their *generation of alternatives* stage in which they view creative idea-finding techniques such as brainstorming and forced relationships as being supported by the research literature (D'Zurilla & Goldfried, pp. 114-117).

Mahoney, in his book *Self-Change* (1979), has identified a model and method for the self-treatment of personal problems such as smoking, obesity, poor work habits and marital difficulties. His approach is, in the main, behavioral and requires a strong motivational set for it to promote positive results. In the stage of his problem-solving model that Mahoney calls *examining possible solutions* he encourages the self-helping problem solver to think of alternative ways of viewing himself and the world (Mahoney, p. 90). Once such alternatives are considered, these alternative beliefs are acted upon in an attempt to change the problem behavior. This part of Mahoney's problem-solving approach requires, then, a creative set, in which the problem solver must think fluently and flexibly.

Jay Haley, from a strategic family therapy approach, has viewed family treatment as problem-solving therapy (Haley, 1978). Haley views such therapy as a creative endeavor. Thinking strategically means that the family therapist must be able to spontaneously and flexibly design interventive procedures for producing change in the client system (Haley, p. 9).

The problem-solving literature has been reviewed by Heppner in an attempt to relate it to the counseling process (1978). Could the counseling process be viewed as a problem-solving event? Heppner concludes that there is enough information to conclude that it could; further he suggests that problem solving in counseling does include the important creative *skill* of successfully generating alternative solutions to the specified problem.

Because generating alternative solutions is a skill, Heppner wants to know how a person can learn or teach such a skill (p. 371). This is a good question, because many of the authors I have cited above have indicated the need for a *creative* problem solving, have discussed in general terms how it might be gotten, *but have failed to concretely specify ways in which it can be promoted*.

Attempts to employ problem solving as a training procedure and as a therapy should be noted. Spivack and Platt, employing a host of problem-solving methods including methods for thinking of alternative solutions to problems with chronic psychiatric patients, found some evidence for change in the patients' ability to think of alternate solutions (1976, p. 372). And an effort at using problem solving in a workshop training format with college students led to improved quality of student responses to problem situations (Dixon et al., 1979, p. 138).

Summary

A review of some of the work related to problem solving in psychology has indicated the following: Based upon literature reviews in the theory and research of problem solving, authors have advocated the use of problem solving as a treatment in behavior modification and for the more general process of counseling. Further, these authors indicate the importance of a creative problem solving by suggesting the use of creative methods for the generation of alternative solutions to the problem. Other authors have suggested the importance of creativity in problem solving; one, Mahoney, from a self-help standpoint encourages it in the client. Haley views creativity as a requirement for the family therapist. And attempts at training and therapy using problem-solving models and methods have used creative methodology as part of these approaches. Creativity has been implicated as a valuable part of the problem-solving process.

THE IMPORTANCE OF CREATIVITY WITHIN A PROBLEM-SOLVING FOCUS

Not only are problem solving and creativity similar processes; it is also apparent that social workers and other professional helpers view creative responses as critical to a successful problem-solving outcome.

A creatively active client problem solver may presume a creative helper. Although we may, as helpers, ask for novel and unique solutions from a client, the likelihood is that many clients without appropriate guidance and training may be simply unable to produce them.

Therefore, we must ask this question: If the helping services are problem-solving focused professions, ones that encourage the use of creativity within a problem-solving approach, then are helping service professionals educated and prepared for a *creative problem solving practice*? Do helpers possess:

> a flexible mind, capable of associating quickly and easily. A richly associating mind, drawing on a wide range of perceptions, making comparisons freely, sensing the general in a mass of particulars, and the particular application of generalities. (Reynolds, 1942, p. 151)

Do helpers possess creative problem-solving abilities? The answer to this question is simply not known. In an attempt to answer this question Klau (1981) reviewed major texts used in graduate schools of social work, course descriptions in graduate school catalogues, dissertation topics, and social work education periodicals to determine whether social work educators emphasized experiential practice in creative problem solving. Klau was not able to find evidence that the educative process, which includes readings, lecture, class discussion and practicum experiences, led to the development of creative problem-solving skills (pp. 36-39). Although the absence of such evidence through the means investigated by Klau does not indicate a deficit in such social work and educational experiences, it does lend some credence to the belief that experience in creative problem solving may be lacking in the social worker's educational background.

Giving further credence to this belief is the evidence that suggests that thinking and problem-solving skills are seldom taught in our colleges and universities (Maeroff, 1983).

THE CREATIVE PRACTITIONER

Donald Schön, in an attempt to counter a stance of *technical rationality* in many of the professions, i.e., a perspective grounded in the belief that problems are best solved by selecting from available means those most qualified to meet established ends, has argued that professionals in today's reality are faced with a practice that does *not* fit the standard problem-solving paradigm (1983, p. 43). Practice, he goes on to say, is not made up of problems that are given, rather they "must be constructed from the materials of problematic situations which are puzzling, troubling and uncertain." A practitioner, therefore, must somehow be capable of making coherent a situation that initially makes no sense at all.

To make sense of seemingly nonsensical situations requires a different kind of problem-solving perspective than that provided by the standard problem-solving model. The practitioner confronted with a client system made up of psychological, social, economic and political issues that present an ambiguous and unique situation must be able to *problem set*. By problem setting, Schön means that capacity to *construct* a problem from a set of uncertain, unclear and unique factors. The practitioner must be able to frame the problem. It is a creative action in that the practitioner must identify those factors that have priority over others and then attend to them in a selected context. The problem selected is an invention, something that prior to the practitioner's attention to it did not exist.

But technical rationality or the practice of a convergent (analytic) model of problem solving does not provide the practitioner with the skills for problem setting. Schein, an organizational development theorist and consultant, contends that there is a difference between the *basic and applied sciences*, which are convergent, i.e., logical, analytical and narrowing in perspective, and *practice*, which is divergent, that is to say, analogical, intuitive and expansive. Because practice has unique and unpredictable elements the practitioner, Schein says, must be able to work with an analytical or convergent knowledge base and convert such knowledge into a practice that is fashioned for the novel elements of various client systems. The practitioner, therefore, must be a creative practitioner. He must use, as Schein says, *divergent thinking skills* (1973, p. 43).

Divergent thinking skills can be defined as those skills that facilitate the production of fluency and flexibility in idea generation. These skills have been identified by Guilford as those used for creative work (1967). Because creativity demands both the generation of novel ideas and their transformation into real-world products a creative problem-solving model must include both divergent and convergent thinking skills. The creative practitioner must invent and then help convert the invention into something useful for helping the client system.

PROBLEM-SOLVING MODELS — PROBLEMS IN THEMSELVES

Most social work authors of texts used for clinical practice, with very few exceptions, either emphasize the importance of a problem-solving approach or provide a descriptive problem-solving model for practice. Important as these guides may be they fall far short of what is required for an effective creative problem-solving practice.[1]

Creative problem-solving practice is important for three reasons:

1. Such practice increases the growth and understanding of the practitioner as he uses the skills inherent in the process to aid others.
2. A creative problem-solving practice encourages the growth of the cognitive and affective capacities of clients previously incapable of employing a problem-solving approach to confront personal-environmental difficulties.
3. Creative problem-solving practice can support the professions need for renewal by encouraging a trend toward social invention. Using creative problem solving can aid in the process of social invention. New procedures, programs and policy may be the result of a creative problem-solving practice.

---

[1]Hepworth and Larsen (1982) provide the main exception to this rule. Their chapter in *Direct Social Work Practice* provides guidelines for a problem-solving practice. However, it must be pointed out that these authors assume that the practitioner is already a fluent, spontaneous and flexible thinker and knows how to promote these qualities in the client (see pp. 319-341).

Meeting these three objectives requires a creative problem-solving model that fulfills at least four conditions:

1. The model must be *descriptive*. It must include a series of steps or stages that must be, at least, partially completed to successfully solve a problem. Such a series of steps indicates that creative problem solving is a *process*.
2. The creative problem-solving model must *identify* the actions that should be carried out in each step of the model. For example, if the model includes a *generation of alternatives* stage, it should indicate what procedures can be used for generating alternatives.
3. The model must clearly *prescribe* the actions that are to be taken by problem solvers in each of its steps. Beyond identifying clearly the procedures to be used, the model should include specific instructions for the problem solver. For example, it is not enough to say that the client must brainstorm alternative solutions, nor is it enough to say that the client should not criticize his ideas as they occur to him. The model should tell us explicitly how brainstorming is employed and how workers and clients can learn to *defer* criticism of their ideas.
4. A creative problem-solving model for helping service practice must also be informed by theories, research and methods from the knowledge domains that have contributed the most to its practice. Psychology, and creative education are those fields that have elaborated on theory and technique for creative problem solving. Theories of creative behaviour; identification of the traits of creative persons through research; a clear understanding of the obstacles to creativity; and an awareness and understanding of the techniques employed in various steps of a *creative* problem-solving model should inform a *creative* problem-solving practice.

In summary, the requirements for a creative problem-solving model for practice to meet the goals of practitioner, client and professional growth can be readily identified. The model must be clear about the *general* operations that are taken in each of its steps. Just as important, it must specify the actions to be taken by problem solvers, and accompanying these action guidelines should be instructions on how to appropriately carry them out. Further, this model must inform us on the knowledge and method coming from various disciplines so as practitioners we understand the basis for problem-solving actions.

A CREATIVE PROBLEM-SOLVING MODEL

A model that meets the conditions listed above is the Parnes model of creative problem solving (1977). This model has been developed from an interplay of practice and research, and has been used to promote creative solutions to problems in industrial technology, business, art and the helping professions. Research of the model has indicated that training in creative problem solving can make an impact on an individual's attitudes and behaviours such as openness to ideas, reducing negative judgment made on ideas and decreasing the inclination to jump to conclusions (Basadur et al., 1982).

The model as presented by Parnes, consists of five stages, these stages divided into two phases. Figure 3 shows the linear stages of the model.

The model comes into play in the following way: the creative problem solver becomes sensitive to some concern, opportunity or challenge that is not understood. The area of concern is fuzzy, vague, ill-defined. Credit must be given to the problem solver for her sensitivity to the concern; this is the first problem-solving action. Responding to a vaguely defined area of concern is a problem-solving skill that can be learned.

Following awareness that a concern exists the problem solver collects facts about the concern and focuses upon the relevant data

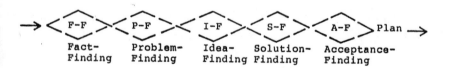

FIGURE 3. The five stages of the Creative Problem-Solving Model.

collected. As can be seen in Table 1 this is a two-phase process called fact-finding and requires two distinct kinds of thinking — *divergent*, scanning and search for data without prejudging the relevance of what is found, and *convergent*, carefully sifting through the data collected for the data most relevant to the concern. I shall say more about these two kinds of thinking in later chapters. Suffice it to say that all stages of CPS consist of this alternation between divergent and convergent thinking.

Focusing upon the relevant data the problem solver produces a number of alternative problem definitions, chooses what she views as a broad representation of the problem and then breaks the problem into workable components.

Then the problem solver generates alternatives for solution. These solutions, at this point, are usually no more than *strategies*, broad directions for change or action. Selection of these strategies is made by producing criteria and selecting those that are best for strategy evaluation. Ideas are now produced for each of the strategies selected. The problem solver again evaluates these ideas by producing, then selecting criteria for evaluation.

Finally, the ideas or idea package is tested by planning for its implementation, then carrying out the plan and evaluating its effects.

The creative problem solver must move through *two* idea-finding stages and *two* solution-finding stages. It is necessary to do so because ideas to a problem are seldom clear, elaborate and concrete in their first form; rather, they are vague, fuzzy, ill-defined and broad plans for change. And that is why I prefer to call them *strategies* when first produced. A further reason for employing two idea-finding stages is that made by D'Zurilla and Goldfried. They state that:

> If the problem solver were to work only at the specific behavior level without first considering strategies, there would be a greater likelihood of "getting into a rut" and staying within only one or a few types of approaches; if these few approaches were not the best for the particular problem in question, effectiveness would be reduced. (1971, p. 117)

TABLE 1. The Creative Problem-Solving Model: Its stages, phases and operations.

Stage	Phase	Operation
Fact-Finding	Divergent	Gather Facts
	Convergent	Select facts most relevant to concern.
Problem-Finding	Divergent	Produce many problem statements from gathered data.
	Convergent	Identify broad statement of problem. Break it down into components. Select one component.
Idea-Finding	Divergent	Generate any alternative solutions to problems as stated.
	Convergent	Identify ideas for possible solution.
Solution-Finding	Divergent	Produce many criteria for use to evaluate and select ideas.
	Convergent	Select most important criteria for use in evaluation and weigh each idea against them. Choose for implementation those ideas that best fit the criteria.
Acceptence-Finding	Divergent	Generate factors that may need to be considered in gaining acceptance for idea.
	Convergent	Steps for action plan are selected and prioritized. Plan is implemented and evaluated. Adjustments based upon evaluation are made.

LINEAR MODELS IN A NON-LINEAR WORLD

The CPS model appears as a series of stages to be followed step-by-step toward the solution of a problem. Unfortunately, that is not the way in which humans think. The following is what John Dewey had to say about his problem-solving model in 1933 and I believe it equally applies to CPS:

> The five phases, terminals or functions of thought that we have noted do not follow one another in a set order. On the contrary, each step in genuine thinking does something to perfect the formation of a suggestion and promote its change into a leading idea or directive hypothesis. It does something to promote the location and definition of the problem. Each improvement in the idea leads to new observations that yield new facts or data and help the mind judge more accurately the relevancy of facts already at hand. The elaboration of the hypothesis does not wait until the problem has been defined and adequate hypothesis has been arrived at; it may come in at any intermediate time. And as we have just seen, any particular overt test need not be final; it may be introductory to new observations and new suggestions, according to what happens in consequence of it. (1933, p. 115)

The CPS model is a tool, then, to be used judiciously for helping service practice and invention. The model should not be *forced* into step-by-step use unless this is dictated by the reality of practice. Human thought is interactive; it cannot only be limited to one function at a time. The problem-solving skills that are indicated in each stage must be learned and internalized so the model may be used flexibly and with spontaneity.

THE MODIFIED CPS MODEL

Figure 4 shows a modified CPS Model. As can be seen it includes seven stages. To use this model the potential problem solver will have to learn more than the names of its stages and the identification of procedures to be taken in each of them. As Haley says of educating family therapists for problem-solving therapy: the thera-

Concern → F-F	P-F	S-F	S-F	I-F	S-F	A-F
Fact-Finding	Problem-Finding	Strategy-Finding	Solution-Finding	Idea-Finding	Solution-Finding	Acceptance-Finding

FIGURE 4. An adaptation of the Osborn-Parnes CPS model.

pist can only learn to do it by doing it (1976, p. 181). That is why part of this book is dedicated to exercises that must be practiced to develop the problem-solving skills necessary for social work practice.

Summary

This chapter has attempted definitions of problem solving and creativity and has found them to be similar processes in many respects. A creative problem-solving process takes place when two conditions exist: (1) when the problem demands a creative response and (2) when the problem solver is able to provide it.

A problem-solving approach with creative attributes has been advocated as a practice approach by social workers and other helping professionals. Further, it has been suggested as an important ingredient in the development of social innovation for social work.

The major thesis of this chapter is that creativity and problem solving can be linked to form a CPS model that is descriptive, identifies actions that practitioners must take, prescribes clearly how the actions should be carried out and draws theory, research and methods from psychology and creative education. This model, the Osborn-Parnes model of CPS, has been modified to include seven stages. The model is valuable because it meets all of the conditions specified for a practice model of creative problem solving. Therefore it can be used to teach helpers and students how to practice a creative problem solving approach.

ADDITIONAL READINGS

J.P. Guilford, Moana Hendricks, and Ralph Hoepfner. "Solving Social Problems Creatively," *Journal of Creative Behavior*, Vol. 2, No. 3, 1968, pp. 155-154.

Helen Harris Perlman, *Social Casework: a problem solving process*. Chicago: The University of Chicago Press, 1957.

Kurt Spitzer and Betty Walsh, "A Problem Focused Model of Practice," *Social Casework*, Vol. 50, No. 6, June, 1969, pp. 323-329.

David Hallowitz, "The Problem-Solving Component in Family Therapy," *Social Casework*, Vol 51, No. 2 Feb., 1970, pp. 67-75.

Darlene V. Howard, *Cognitive Psychology: memory, language and thought*. New York: MacMillan Publishing Co., 1983, Chapter 12, Problem Solving.

EXERCISE

One thing educators frequently warn us about is getting ahead of ourselves. Because this is a book about creative problem solving it is appropriate that we reverse this admonition. Let's get ahead of ourselves. Let's do this by predicting what kind of skills creative problem solving requires. Start getting ahead by following these guidelines:

1. Form into groups of 5-7 individuals. Make sure everyone knows each other by their first name. Appoint a group recorder.
2. Consider the following guideline before beginning to predict the skills required for creative problem solving—*allow yourself to say anything you want to say in the group without criticizing yourself, further, don't criticize anything said by any group member no matter how unusual; or unfeasible it may sound to you* (in other words, don't criticize anything said by yourself or others).
3. Produce (name) as many problem-solving skills as you believe are necessary for creative problem solving within a five minute time period.
4. When the time period is up all participating groups should put each of their ideas on a small piece of paper or a card. Tape the papers or cards to the room walls with masking tape.
5. All group participants should then move about the room, look-

ing carefully at all the ideas on the papers or cards. Each participant should vote for *three* ideas (skills) they consider to be most important for creative problem solving. Vote by starring or checking with crayon or pencil the appropriate skill.

6. Identify those skills most favoured by the total group. List them in a place easily observable to all.

7. Discuss each skill so that: (1) all group participants are clear about its meaning and (2) why it is considered to be important for creative problem solving.

Chapter 2

Explaining Creativity

Understanding how theorists have viewed creativity may help the creative problem solver. Meichenbaum has demonstrated the use of creativity theory by operationalizing the major ideas embedded in them, and in so doing has shown that creativity can be enhanced by changing what individuals say to themselves about these operationalized theoretical ideas (1975).

There have been numerous attempts to theoretically explain creativity. At the risk of oversimplifying, however, these theories can be sorted into three major groupings. One group of theories is marked by the idea that creativity can be explained by the *mental skills* individuals possess. Prominent among this group of thinkers is J. P. Guilford (1977). Guilford has developed the Structure-of-Intellect model of intelligence; within this model he has assigned divergent thinking as the motor for producing creative thought. As Guilford says:

> The greatest importance of divergent-production abilities is in connection with creative thinking, where many alternative ideas need to be brought to light with ease. Since creative thinking is an important aspect of problem solving, these abilities are also important in that connection. (1977, p. 108)

Guilford makes the link between creative thinking and problem-solving behavior. When a unique problem is faced we must call up many possible solutions through our capacity for divergent thinking.

A second grouping of theories of creativity can be compiled under the rubric of *psychiatry*. Beginning with Freud, the father of

psychoanalysis, a number of psychoanalytically and psychiatri-
cally-trained thinkers have attempted to understand creative phenomena. Freud, Kris and Arieti are some of the names associated
with this theoretical group.

A third group of creativity theories exists. These thinkers emphasize the *personality and attitudinal* factors involved in creative behavior. The work of Donald MacKinnon (1962) and his associates
have contributed to this school of thought.

Fortunately, many of the ideas about creativity that these three
groups put forward have *some* use and can be made to work in
practice. Some of the ideas, as we will see, are better substantiated
by research than others.

What I hope to demonstrate in this chapter is:

1. at present there are a *number* of different theories that attempt
   to explain creativity;
2. that it is important to be familiar with these theoretical ideas so
   they can provide a theoretical foundation for a creative problem-solving model, and
3. that although these ideas appear to be, at first glance, mutually
   exclusive, they can be used in conjunction with each other.

MENTAL ABILITIES AND CREATIVITY

Divergent thinking, Guilford says, is the ability to search broadly
for many facts, problems, ideas and evaluative criteria when faced
with a problem situation (1977, p. 92). The divergent thinker has
several important characteristics. First, she is *fluent*. This is the
ability to quickly produce many of whatever is necessary to meet
the demand of the problem situation. For example, a poet searches
for a better word to evoke the mood she is attempting to convey. In
order to find this word she searches through her mind for those
words that have definitional equivalence. Mozart was a fluent com-
poser, able to complete works such as the overture to Don
Giovanni, the story goes, the night previous to its first playing
(Perkins, p. 164).

Not only must a divergent thinker be fluent, Guilford says, but
she also must have *flexibility of thought* (1977, p. 167). By flexibil-

ity of thought is meant the ability to shift ideas and objects to various categories. Let's take the example of a helping service worker who is attempting to produce ideas about the problem of a wife confronted with an abusive husband. Below is an actual list of ideas produced by a helping service student prior to practice in becoming flexible in thinking:

- list change in her routine
- list any change in husband's routine
- list occasions when husband gets angry
- list what they were doing when angry
- list what he was doing when angry
- get a divorce
- try separation

As you can see many of the ideas fall into the same class; the ideas are similar, related to noticing by listing changes in behavior. Although the student gets credit for producing seven ideas the ideas cannot, except in a few cases, be considered highly distinguishable from each other.

Let's look at a sample of this student's ideas after one semester in a creative problem-solving course. A different problem but one judged equivalent in difficulty is presented to the student — that of a married man with three children who has been passed over for the promotion he very much wanted. (See Figure 5.)

- re-evaluate how well he has done on the job
- talk to family for reassurance
- become active in areas of interest
- evaluate why other worker got the job
- take time to decide next job move
- re-establish life with wife
- continue giving high performance
- ask boss how he thinks he might get promotion
- talk with friends about reasons why he may have failed

This student has escaped premature "hardening of the categories." By learning to shift from class to class she now exemplifies a flexible thinker.

DIVERGENT THINKING

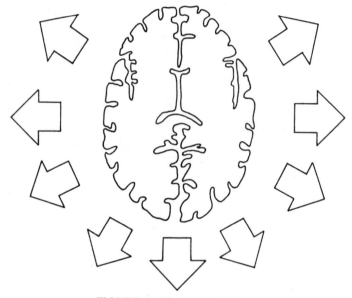

FIGURE 5. Divergent thinking.

D. N. Perkins (1981) is another theorist who believes strongly in the importance of mental abilities for creative work. He states that the mind of the inventive individual works similarly to the mind of the non-inventive person. Just as the athlete is someone who is stronger, more coordinated and more fit than we are, the creative person is one who can remember more, and more efficiently, notices more about himself and his environment, and realizes more than his non-creative counterpart.

Perkins assaults a number of creative positions. For example, he calls the belief ideas coming to us after a long period of unconscious work the still-waters theory. (See Figure 6.) This theory can be discounted, he says, if we look deeply into the self-reports of such great thinkers as Wallace and Darwin. In their cases, the work of evolutionary theory was not illuminated from the unconscious;

rather, Perkins says, it proceeded step-by-step, with one sequence of thought heading on to the next.

Perkins also takes exception to Blitzkrieg theory, and attempts to explain it by invoking normal mental mechanisms. Blitzkrieg theory, he says, is that notion that we can explain extraordinary insights or "mental leaps" by an accelerated thought process that compresses considerable normal mental effort into a few seconds (1981, p. 58). Moving from one point in our thinking to the next rapidly, Perkins notes, can be explained by the act of *recognition* rather than an unexplainably rapid thought process. If, as helping service workers, we have faced a number of client situations that have similar features we can *quickly* recognize these features; we quickly identify the pattern of the situation as the same as others. Problems that require insight to solve are done so by *realizing*, the act of abrupt understanding. And abrupt understanding or gaining an insight is quite different from mysteriously experiencing a brainstorm as contended by Blitzkrieg theorists. (See Figure 7.) The client, who in a therapeutic situation gains an insight, or who realizes

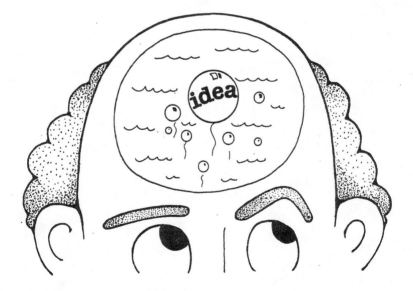

FIGURE 6. Still-Waters theory.

something highly important to her life situation, has worked through much previous material in getting to this point. The feeling that attends the insight, that of excitement or satisfaction, is related to the achievement of it, and not necessarily to any rapid or accelerated thought process.

Guilford and Perkins are two creativity theorists that focus upon the cognitive factors involved in the creative process. They view the creative individual as using basic mental operations to solve problems — divergent thinking and its attendant skills of fluency and flexibility in the case of Guilford, and remembering, noticing, recognizing and realizing in Perkins's view. We can see that although both count heavily on mental abilities, those that they identify for creative work are different. Guilford places his understanding of creativity upon the thinker who searches for many ideas that tend to fall in varied categories. Perkins views creativity as involving mundane, rather commonplace mental activities. The creative thinker uses much the same mental activities that all of us use but with the additional proposition that he basically remembers, recognizes and realizes *more* than the non-creative individual.

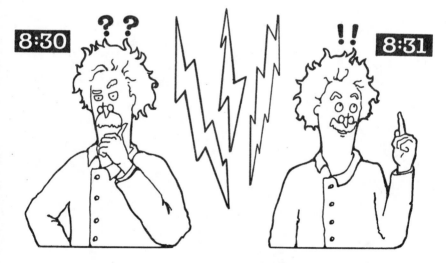

FIGURE 7. Blitzkrieg theory.

PSYCHIATRIC THEORIES

Psychoanalysis, through its founder and several of its followers, has attempted to shed light on the creative phenomenon.

Freud, the founder of the psychoanalytic movement in psychiatry, in his early thought, linked creative writing with fantasy (1959a). He believed that poets and novelists use actual experiences in the present to stimulate memories of early experiences, usually from childhood, and re-work both the actual and remembered experiences into wishful (fantastic) thought. The re-worked material becomes the stuff of plays, poems and novels.

In a later theoretic statement Freud viewed creativity as a reconciliation between reality and fantasy (1959b). Artists use fantasy to find their way back to reality. Using their considerable talents they mold their fantasies into creative products that are accorded value and respect by society.

Kris, from his vantage point as an ego psychoanalyst, suggested that the artist could voluntarily exercise a relaxation of control of the ego. The artist could purposefully regress to make contact with preconscious and unconscious material helpful in creating (1954).

Arieti, in his book *Creativity: the magic synthesis*, has attempted a comprehensive explanation of the creative process in psychiatric terms (1976). In it Arieti identifies a number of different mechanisms that are used in producing creativity.

The *image*, he says, is a useful tool for creative thinking. By imaging Arieti means that we are using "our mind's eye." We are able to visualize persons, objects, or experiences that may not actually exist in the present. As example, close your eyes and imagine your mother. Although she is not present her image is with you; this image represents her. Imaging can occur in other sensory modalities beyond the visual. Some individuals can reproduce sounds and conversation from their experience; others can taste different foods without the food stimulus.

How does the image contribute to creative thinking? The image as Arieti has defined it is a purely mental occurrence. It attempts to represent something from our storehouse of experience. But an image, say of our mother, cannot be accurately reproduced. And this fact frees us from a totally accurate reproduction of our reality. In producing images, Arieti says, we distort them. The image, then, is a way of creating. As we image we make modifications of reality, embellishing parts of objects, persons, or experiences in our idiosyncratic way. Images can add or subtract from reality. What we experience in "our mind's eye" is an approximation and substitute for reality.

Images can help us create in many ways. Let me mention one. When we image, we image not only a person, place or thing but connected with the images are a set of feelings, some related to the image from the past and some coming from our present evaluation of it. These feelings shape and form the image. The artist, for example, may be drawing the body of a nude. In the act of drawing many images may interpose themselves between the artist's perception of the nude. The feelings attached to these images may change the artist's rendering of the nude in creative ways. The changes that the image-feeling unit make on the perception are what artists call their *style* of drawing. Later we will see how images can help us solve helping service problems. Not only can images be used to get solutions, images can help us incubate so solutions to problems may come forth more readily.

Another mechanism that Arieti identifies for creative production is *paleologic*. In an earlier work Arieti had suggested that such thought was the kind that characterized schizophrenia (1955). Paleologic, Arieti maintains, is a primitive form of thought and differs from Aristotelian logic in that it is based upon *identification of predicates*. Individuals using paleologic thought identify persons, objects or experiences as equal because, *in some respect*, they are *similar*.

Arieti gives the example of the schizophrenic woman who thought she was the Virgin Mary. When asked why she thought so, she replied, "I am a virgin. The Virgin Mary was a virgin; I am the Virgin Mary." What the psychotic woman has done is draw an attribute from herself and another, and on the basis of this sameness claimed an equivalence with the other person. Another example: a psychotic person claims to be sucking on his mother's breast while eating an apple. Because the apple and the breast have a similar quality, that of roundness, the psychotic, using paleologic, draws the conclusion that the apple and the breast are the same.

Why can paleologic, allied as it is with the schizophrenic, lead to creative thinking? It is so because paleologic diverges from our logical thought processes and helps us consider different perspectives. As a poet we may look for metaphors and similes which are formed when we identify similarities between the attributes of different things or processes. For example — "A beagle's tail, sickle-shaped, slices the air, as dog sniffs and moves from tree to bush to tree." The poet identifies the crescent shape of the dog's tail with that of a sickle. A spinning top may be identified with the earth; the raging ocean with the fury of our emotions; our significance throughout human history, with a speck of sand.

The ability to notice parts of processes or things that are similar to others may lead to inventions. By watching a shipworm burrowing into a timber Sir March Isumbard Brunel solved the problem of underwater construction. By observing the worm constructing a tube for itself as it moved forward, Brunel came to the idea of caissons (Gordon, 1961). Papanek has coined the word "Bionics" to stand for the field that uses such observations drawn from biological and physical processes for use in invention (1969).

Can paleologic be used for the helping services? Yes, paleologic has been used by Gordon to develop the method for creative production of Synectics. In Chapter 7 we will use Synectics to help us solve helping service problems.

In summary I have discussed the theoretic contributions of Freud, Kris and Arieti. Freud has emphasized the use of fantasy for creative production. Kris has amplified on Freud's idea by suggesting the way to fantasy is through a purposeful relaxation of ego controls and functions — a regression. Arieti contends that images, akin to fantasy and capable of evoking them, are sources of creative productivity due to the way they distort original perceptions leading to various ways of seeing persons, processes and objects. Paleologic, or archaic thought, can be used in the creative process because it leads to divergence. Purposeful paleological thought may provide us with insights from analogies and metaphors. Such insights may contribute to invention.

NON-INTELLECTIVE THEORIES OF CREATIVITY

A third group of creative theories have been built around the thesis that there are personality and attitudinal differences between creative and non-creative persons. Barron clearly states this thesis when he suggests that if:

> some persons are regularly original, whereas others are regularly unoriginal, it must be the case that certain patterns of relatively enduring traits either facilitate or impede the production of original acts. (1955, p. 478)

Writers such as Barron (1955), Rogers (1962), McMullan (1976) and MacKinnon (1965) have attempted to identify the qualities that are associated with individual creative production.

Barron's research is indicative of this theoretical approach. He looks for those qualities associated with the *original* person. By original Barron means two things. One, that originality must be defined as an act that is relatively uncommon in a particular group. An original response is a statistically infrequent response. Secondly, an original response must relate to reality; it must be of some use in problem solving.

Barron (1955) has found that the original and non-original person can be differentiated based upon the following factors:

1. originals prefer complexity and some degree of assymetry in phenomena
2. original persons depend less upon outside evaluation; they are more independent than non-originals in their judgement
3. originals are less likely to suppress impulses that are considered taboo than are non-originals. Originals dislike to police themselves or others
4. original persons possess more self-assertion than non-originals

It is interesting to note Carl Rogers's (1962) theory of creativity as it relates to Barron's findings about the original person. Rogers suggests three factors that the individual must have for creative work. The creative person, he says, must be *open to experience*. No matter the origin of stimuli, either environmental or of an internal nature, the person, to make use of these stimuli, must perceive them without distortion. According to Rogers the creative individual is *non-defensive*. An artist, for example, would not reject frightening fantasy or dream material but would record it perceptually and use it in the artistic product. By accepting them as part of himself and by using them, such internal productions are transformed. Helping service workers have learned that the self, perceiving and responding non-defensively to the moment-to-moment reality of clients, is the instrument that aids clients in finding their own undistorted reality (Shulman, 1979, p. 42). Rogers identifies a second quality that an individual must have to possess creativity—*an internal locus of evaluation*. By this he means that whatever is made by the individual has been based on her evaluation of the product and not by the praise or criticism of others. What has been created must be satisfying to the individual: the creation must express some part of this person in action. If the creative product has satisfied the requirement that it represents such self-expression, it is perceived so by the individual. No outside evaluation can change this fact. This does not mean that the creating person does not accept *any* criticism; rather, it means that such evaluation is not the primary source of satisfaction as related to the product.

Do the helping services recognize the value of an internal locus of evaluation? The helping professions have considered the *non-judgmental attitude* to be a major principle in helping others (Biestek, 1957). In practice non-judgmental attitude should work by allowing clients who receive this attitude to explore themselves. The freedom to find undiscovered parts of themselves is permitted by such an attitude. By experiencing the previously undiscovered parts of their selves clients begin to prize these parts. Such a process tends to reinforce the idea that the self should be the locus of evaluation.

A third factor that Rogers identifies as a requirement for creativity is the ability *to play with elements and concepts*. Ideas, shapes, colors, relationships between concepts, etc., are considered to be those things that can be explored and spontaneously experimented upon. In this manner the person may find a new and significant way to solve a problem.

There is considerable dovetailing between Rogers's creativity theory and Barron's research findings. The notion of an internal locus of evaluation is reinforced by Barron's finding that original persons depend less upon outside evaluation. Rogers's idea that creative persons must be playful is supported in part by Barron's finding that originals are less likely to suppress impulses that are considered unconventional or taboo than do non-originals. Such a finding would suggest that such impulses are at the original's command for spontaneous exploration.

CREATIVE INDIVIDUALS: PARADOXICAL PERSONAGES

McMullan (1976) has formulated a theory of the creative person by noticing a number of personality traits of creatives that, at first glance, apparently contradict each other. He notes, for example, that theorists have described the requisites of creativity as (1) the *trait of flexibility*, or capacity to spontaneously play, and (2) the *quality of persistence*, whereby an idea is made feasible through hard work and discipline. How can these two notions of creative persons be reconciled? McMullan suggests that this seeming paradox, the capacity of creative persons to be both playful and hardworking is the core characteristic of the creative individual. Creative persons are, according to McMullan, to be described as *flexibly persistent*. Surrounding this core is set a number of other apparently contradictory traits. Figure 8 shows the complete set of paradoxical qualities that McMullan believes describes the various aspects of the creative person.

What McMullan has done is synthesized the work of a number of creativity theorists in an attempt to resolve the conflicting sets of traits attributed to the creative person. One example of such contradiction is the portrayal of the creative person as both confident and humble (self-concept). Several authors have concluded that confidence is a generally accepted characteristic of creative individuals (Dellas & Gaier, 1970; Whitfield, 1975). On the other hand McMullan cites Maslow (1971) who has defined the creative person as one who perceives the world with awe, fascination and innocence, an admission of his smallness in the face of the world's complexity. Maslow believes that this is the form humility takes in the creative.

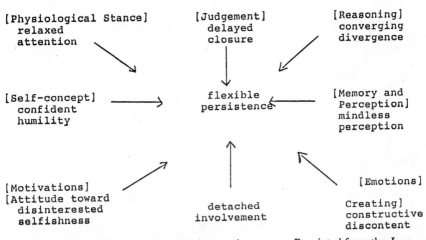

FIGURE 8. Paradoxical qualities of the creative person. Reprinted from the *Journal of Creative Behavior* by permission of the publishers, Creative Education Foundation, Buffalo, New York, © 1977.

The creative person, McMullan says, resolves this contradiction in traits by using each of the seemingly conflicting traits for a specific creative problem-solving purpose. The humility of the creative allows him to be *flexible*, to admit doubt, to be skeptical of findings, and to question work critically. Confidence is used for *persistence*. While doubtful of the work at hand, the creative individual tenaciously moves ahead with it, aware all the while of its possible inadequacy.

McMullan has ordered the eight pairs of paradoxical traits by separating them into a flexibility and persistent set (Figure 9). The flexibility set of traits is used to find ideas; whereas the persistence set is employed to elaborate and evaluate. What McMullan has constructed is a two-step conceptualization of creativity that connects with our model of CPS as outlined in Chapter 1.

Remember that in all stages of CPS are a divergent and convergent phase. The divergent phase employs the traits as McMullan identifies them in the flexibility set to search and explore. The flexibility set serves the total personality in such a search. The convergent phase, however, makes use of the persistence set to elaborate upon the fruits of the divergent search. Evaluation and planning is

flexibility set	persistence set
humble self-concept	confident self-concept
disinterested motivation	selfish motivation
discontented attitude	constructive attitude
mindless perception	understanding based on memory
divergent thought	convergent thought
relaxation	attention
delay in closure	systematic closure
emotional involvement	emotional detachment

FIGURE 9. Ordering of eight paradoxical sets of personality traits under the core characteristics of the creative person.

done to implement ideas found in the divergent phase. McMullan's conception of creativity can be perceived as a problem-solving process, whereby the problem-solver oscillates between the flexibility and persistence sets, using first one set, then the other, in a progression toward problem resolution.

Summary

This chapter has provided a view of the three main bodies of theory that attempt to explain creativity. Mental ability, psychiatric and personality approaches to creativity have been presented.

It probably has occurred to you as you have read this chapter that these different bodies of theory overlap. Although Arieti comes from a psychiatric tradition his creative mechanisms, viz., the image, and paleologic thinking might have been considered as mental abilities. Perkins, although he stresses the cognitive aspects of creativity, is reluctant to rule out personal-attitudinal factors in the creative process (1981, pp. 269-274).

How helpful is it for us to be familiar with these theories? Each type of theory has led to the development of techniques useful in creative thinking and problem solving. From the mental abilities approach have come idea-finding techniques used to produce divergent thinking and its attendant qualities of fluency and flexibility. The psychiatric school has influenced interest in contacting mental processes below the level of conscious awareness. Relaxation and incubation techniques are ways used to make such a connection.

The personality theories of creativity have encouraged an expansion of the self through greater self-awareness. These theories, then, indicate pathways to be taken to improve the creativity of the individual. The value of a theory of creativity resides, for the purposes of creative problem solving, in our ability to employ its key elements in creative action. Our ability to operationalize a theoretical concept makes it a valuable instrument for seeking creative ideas.

ADDITIONAL READINGS

Frank Barron. *Creativity and Personal Freedom*. Princeton, N.J.: Van Nostrand, 1968.

Albert Rothenberg. *The Emerging Goddess: The Creative Process in Art, Science and other Fields*. Chicago: University of Chicago Press, 1979.

Ann Roe. "A Psychological Study of Eminent Biologists" *Psychological Monographs*, Vol. 65, No. 14, 1951.

Jerome S. Bruner. Beyond the Information Given. New York: Norton, 1973.

Hans J. Eysenck. "The Roots of Creativity: Cognitive Ability or Personality Trait?" Roeper Review, Vol. 5, No. 4, April-May, 1983.

EXERCISE – THEORY CONSTRUCTION

Can you develop your own theory of creativity? Remember, Rogers has hypothesized that creative people are able to play with concepts and elements so that new arrangements may be found. Therefore, I am issuing you a challenge. Can you theorize?

Here are some tips for developing your theory of creativity:

— Think about any creative person you know. What is it about them that you think facilitates their creativity?
— Have you observed creative persons thinking? How do they think?
— Notice completed creative products such as paintings, sculptures, inventions, films, excellent meals, etc. What do you imagine were the ways the creative person went about producing them?

— Ask yourself questions about creativity, the creative person and the creative product. Start with who? what? where? why? how? and when? and ask any question you wish. Try to answer these questions to your satisfaction. Find the answers, if you can, by using books or questioning experts accessible to you.

— With the data you have compiled, write down a number of statements you believe to be true about creativity, the creative person or the creative product. These statements comprise the beginning of a theory. These statements are hypotheses that require testing but, at the very least, are grounded in your and others' experience.

— Look over your statements about creativity. Are there any two statements that relate to each other? See if you can join them. Relationship between your statements may lead to further understanding of the ideas you are considering.

Use the space below to construct your theory.

_____

_____

_____

_____

_____

_____

_____

_____

_____

_____

_____

_____

Chapter 3

Blocks to Creative Problem Solving

Why is it difficult to be original? Why is creativity a phenomenon so infrequently seen? The most fundamental answer to these questions is that most of us experience blocks that *we* or *someone* have placed in our creative problem-solving path. We are confronted with obstacles that must be overcome if we are to create.

Perhaps the simplest way to illustrate how obstacles function to stifle alternative or divergent behavior is to take the example of arm folding. Each of us has a characteristic way of folding our arms in front of us. I, for example, cross my right arm over my left, tucking my right hand between my body and the right bicep and placing my left hand on the side of my left bicep. Whatever way you fold your arm, try now to fold them the opposite of the way you usually do. How do you feel? Strange, I'll bet. When we try to go against habit our initial reaction frequently is discomfort. And when we try to break mental habits of long standing we experience similar feelings of stress and discomfort. Thinking about concerns and problems in established ways, or using solutions that have worked in the past, even though there may be a better way of solving the problem, is a form of rigidity. This type of rigidity is called *response set* because it involves a continual use of a response that was effective in other situations.

There are other blocks to creative problem-solving behavior. As we look at these blocks we see that they can be categorized as *psychological*, *socioeconomic* and *characterological* in nature.

PSYCHOLOGICAL BLOCKS

Throughout childhood many of us are exposed to experiences that indicate that the way we perform is not what others expect of us. We may learn from such experiences that there is a right and wrong way of doing things, thus limiting our response repertoires. From parents, teachers and other authority figures in our milieu, we learn that habit and custom is behavior that is best to follow. Because of this kind of learning we raise our *risk threshold*. Rather than take a reasonable risk when confronted with something new we may tend to "play it safe." We do things the way they have always been done. We become rigid because we dare not risk.

Not only may we shy away from risk because of early conditioning we also become *afraid to fail*. Raising our risk threshold and fear of failure are, of course, interconnected. If I fear failure I certainly will not risk. Alternatively if I am unwilling to risk I develop fear of failure when confronted with situations that require risk. Not having the experience of both succeeding and failing creates a heightened fear of the unknown. Why should I try to think of new ways to develop a group program for unmarried mothers? Even if the program that we have isn't working that well it's better than trying something that might possibly backfire. Individuals with a heightened fear of failure experience feelings of inadequacy, anxiety and embarrassment upon failure. But failure does not have to lead to these kinds of feelings. If failure can be viewed as an inevitable part of life the experience of it can be used as an instructive lesson for the future.

Recently, I made a videotape that illustrated the creative problem-solving process. I had never made a videotape before. Before I began the project I experienced feelings of anxiety and inadequacy. I couldn't begin the project. I was paralyzed—I couldn't take action. Anxious and doubtful I came close to chucking the whole project. And then I began to think of the positive aspects of such an undertaking. Couldn't I learn the mechanics of the videotape-making process? Couldn't I learn how editing is done? I could learn many new skills by doing the project. My anxiety and fear turned to excitement as I thought of what lay in store for me by taking the risk of this project.

Abraham Maslow (1962) identifies several emotional blocks to creativity. He cites the rigid, or obsessive-compulsive personality as being a major obstacle to the creative life. Maslow does not deny that many persons with these personality traits exhibit what he calls *secondary creativity*, that which proceeds exclusively from logical and analytical thought. Therefore the rigid personality might make a good journeyman scientist developing new knowledge in an orderly and systematic fashion. Maslow believed that this kind of personality could not admit anything new into their thinking that would produce a highly creative response.

Maslow noted, too, that as we grow up we turn away from parts of ourselves that do not fit with our culture's definition of gender. If we are male we tend to deny our femaleness, as society defines it. Females reject their socially-defined masculine traits. We can imagine what damage is done by these rejections of opposite-sexed traits. If male we might reject imagination, fantasy, color, poetry, music, tenderness and languishing. Conversely, females might tend to deny their tough-mindedness, competitiveness, athletic ability, scientific capacities, etc. MacKinnon's research with creative architects has shown that they display a high degree of interest in activities considered by the culture to be feminine (1977). It stands to reason that creative persons first view themselves as *persons* rather than male or female. By using everything we are given we have a much better chance of exercising our creativity.

Another block to creativity is what Alamshah (1972) calls our *attitude toward talent*. We can, on the one hand, underestimate the importance for talent in creative work; on the other hand we can overemphasize or exaggerate its significance for creativity.

When talent is underestimated we may notice it in a person's behavior in two ways. First, there is the person who doggedly pursues a vocation for which they are completely ill-suited. For example, consider the individual who goes into the helping service without possessing empathy or caring for people. This person is underestimating the talent required for creative work in this field. Another way talent is underestimated is illustrated through the Peter Principle. Frequently we see helping service workers who have worked in direct practice moved up to supervisory or other administrative positions based upon their direct practice competence. Creative at one kind of helping service they may decidedly lack the kinds of talents and abilities to work creatively at their new position.

How can an exaggerated notion of the importance of talent block creativity. The individual who believes talent to be all-important does not consider the other factors noted by researchers in the creative process—such traits and attitudes as persistence, independence, open-mindedness and the like. These factors should be taken seriously because we see their importance for creative production. Thus, talent cannot be all-important. Exaggerating talent may block creativity also when talented individuals fail to realize that talent by itself cannot produce creativity. Knowledge, judgement and practice are necessary for its development.

In summary: I have discussed some *psychological* obstacles that prevent creative behavior. Fear of failure, and unwillingness to risk, emotional rigidity, fear of our opposite-gender traits, and our attitude toward talent all can play a part in making us less than creative.

CHARACTEROLOGICAL BLOCKS

Alamshah (1972) has defined a characterological blockage to creativity as something lacking in our *inner* development that prevents creative behavior. These blocks are deficiencies of character in the common sense and moral view of character.

A major character defect is that of lack of *self-discipline*. Without it the talent that we possess cannot be harnessed for creative work. Much of the early educative process is an attempt to help us develop discipline. Perkins (1981) has indicated that self-discipline is as important for invention as talent and purpose. He believes that it is the talented and self-directed person, who makes Herculean demands upon the self, that will invent. Therefore, lack of self-discipline, the inability to make such demands upon the self, is not a character flaw we expect in creative persons.

Another significant characterological block is the focus upon *external* rather than *internal* rewards. If our goals are to be rich and recognized and famous they may stand in the way of acting creatively. Frequently, we see in our society many examples of this emphasis upon the external rewards, rewards that come from a minor creative talent. Celebrities—movie and rock stars, for example—may judge their work exclusively upon the external rewards they reap without consulting their internal locus of evaluation. Authors, who write in a highly popular vein, may work quickly without evaluating the creative worth of their work and may just as rapidly fade from the cultural milieu. What is required of the creative is an *involvement with the process* of the work itself. Satisfaction must be gained from the work in progress rather than only from the end product. Barbara McClintock, when learning that she had received the Nobel prize for her work on "jumping genes" said she never wished for such recognition, rather only the respect of her colleagues (1983). Maslow in his study of self-actualizing persons has identified the *problem-centering* quality of these individuals (1970). By this he means that they see their chosen work as something they *must* do rather than want to do. It is unselfish work, centered outside of themselves for the benefit of others or society in general.

SOCIOECONOMIC BLOCKS

Along with psychological and characterologic blocks the potentially creative person can also be faced with blocks coming from socioeconomic sources.

A most significant obstacle to creativity can come from society itself. Our society asks of each individual that he contribute to its maintenance. Tumin (1962, p. 107) has noted that "the attitude of society at large . . . , so far as any individual member is concerned, is primarily instrumental." We must find a useful place in the social order if we are to gain reward and some measure of recognition. As helping service workers this may mean that we must fit effectively into the bureaucratic structure of a social agency. We must do useful work without deviating significantly from the role assigned to us. This is the way, Tumin says, we receive our status in society; this status that we derive from the instrumental work we do makes us feel safe and secure.

It follows, then, that if we ask others, for example, young persons, to try their hand at creative activity we are facing a formidable obstacle in our attempts to help them. For young people have very little status, hence safety, in our society. They seldom hold meaningful jobs, nor have they, because of the way our economic system is now run, had much opportunity to hold meaningful jobs during their adolescent years.

I like the role, then, that Tumin assigns the educator in helping others overcome this societal block to creativity. It is the role of *social reformer*. The teacher who values creativity and problem-solving must help students and other persons recognize that status-striving stands strongly in the way of creative life. The society that pays only modest attention to status should in the long run place less societal constraints upon creative expression than the society in which status is highly regarded.

Related to status-striving as an obstacle to creativity is the emphasis that society places upon a specific and *narrow* conception of human intelligence. Educators reinforce *conceptual* thinking in our schools. From a very early age we learn to think analytically and causally. This kind of thinking is important, for it has undergirded the Western scientific tradition. But if other types of thinking related to other kinds of cognitive styles are disregarded we are bound for trouble. What our schools disregard, in the main, is *social* and *aesthetic* intelligence.

Social intelligence embraces that set of attitudes and skills that is useful in human relationships. It emphasizes the importance of concern and caring for others, individually and in groups. It focuses upon cooperation rather than conflict but it also considers conflict by offering ways to reduce it. Social intelligence embraces those skills relevant for making good decisions and developing reasonable goals by using an acceptable and appropriate set of human values.

Aesthetic intelligence is used in all human endeavors that consider beauty, proportion and design. How do we design an environment appropriate to the needs of the elderly? What are the important considerations to be made when designing a house? How should a playground be planned? What colors should be used to facilitate good working conditions? All of these questions should be placed before those who possess aesthetic intellectual capacity.

If educators only consider conceptual intelligence, while disregarding social and aesthetic intellectual styles of thinking, there is strong chance that some that are so taught will develop blockages if only by way of deficiencies in learning.

There is evidence that helping service workers possess a belief system that maintains that social intelligence, although important, should not be taught or learned in professional schools. Cole and Lacefield (1980) surveyed a number of professional helping service fields, of which social work was one. Those surveyed believed that although affective education, the education of feelings and emotions, was an important component of professional education, it should not be included in these professional curricula.

Another socioeconomic block that should be discussed is the unavailability of *cultural and/or physical resources* to the potentially creative individual (Arieti, 1976). Clearly, if we are poverty-stricken we will have very little chance to express creativity. The cliché of the starving artist aside, there are few poor persons who circumvent this obstacle and reach creative heights. If we are poor we are likely to be under- or poorly educated. And without adequate education there is little chance of expressing creativity. Creativity, as Wallas recognized, requires an intense period of preparation (1926).

Frequently, creativity is not actualized because a culture has not progressed technologically to the point where it can suit or fill the needs of the creatively advanced individual. In other words the creative idea is sound but the technological means to reach it are not available. Leonardo da Vinci's work on the submarine and airplane come to mind. It has been established that there is a time lag between the production of a creative idea and its use by society (Deutsch et al., 1971). Although this lag occurs for many reasons, one of them frequently is society's inability to provide the technical means to actualize the idea. Consider the concept of empathy as it worked its way into the helping service literature in the 1970s. The idea was taken by Carl Rogers in the middle 1950s; he made empathy a major concept in his theory of therapeutic change (1957). From there Truax and Carkhuff researched the concept and developed the technological means to transmit the skills to helpers

(1967). Slowly the theory and the technology that stemmed from it entered the mainstream of helping service thought. Only when the technology was there in teachable form did the helping service professions respond to the empathy concept in a meaningful way.

One last socioeconomic obstacle I would like to discuss is the receptivity of the social milieu to the creative person. Can creative persons express themselves in work situations where creative expression is not expected? The environment I have in mind is one where there is a focus on "going along to get along." This situation is marked by a high degree of decision-making reached through group consensus. Problem-solving discussions are frequently characterized by criticism and evaluation, thereby limiting exchange of ideas. Creative persons do not do well in these situations. Because these persons see ideas initially as equivalent in value, an environment that constantly evaluates an idea before it has time to germinate is viewed as frustrating and destructive to the creative problem-solving process (Prince, 1970).

Blockages to creativity fall, in the main, into psychological, characterological and socioeconomic categories. It is important to identify and understand these obstacles and then determine whether any of them belong to us. Our fear of failure, if not conquered, for example, may block all of our attempts to express creativity.

Can we do something to overcome these obstacles? Certainly the first step in helping oneself is to be *aware* that we have a block. Then we must decide how we can reduce its effect upon us.

Do helping service students have blocks to creativity? I asked a fourth year undergraduate class in Creative Problem-Solving to identify, through the use of an idea-getting technique, the blocks to creativity they considered most difficult to solve. The class of 25 students produced over 120 different kinds of blocks and then evaluated them for significance. Below is a list of these blocks in order of perceived difficulty.

- fear of failure
- lack of self-confidence
- lack of self-discipline
- conformity to social norms
- anxiety

Fear of failure, lack of self-confidence, lack of self-discipline and conformity to social norms were those mentioned most frequently by this class.

Do working adults possess blocks to creativity that are very different than our helping service students? Not really. Using the same idea-getting technique as employed with the students, I asked an adult education class to list their major blocks to creativity. They identified as most difficult:

— fear of failure
— conformity to social norms
— inability to produce alternative ideas
— lack of self-discipline
— inability to cope with daily activities

So we see that fear of failure, social conformity and lack of self-discipline are common blocks to the helping service and adult education groups. Whether these obstacles are those that would be named by other groups cannot be said with any certainty. But I believe that there is significance in the fact that these three blocks were identified by both groups as high in perceived difficulty. It is apparent that before we can be creative we must try to resolve some of these obstacles that stand in the way of our creativity.

ADDITIONAL READINGS

James L. Adams. Conceptual Blockbusting: a guide to better ideas. San Francisco: W.H. Freeman and Co., 1974.
Ellen Y. Siegelman. Personal Risk: mastering change in love and work. New York: Harper and Row, 1983.
Robert Birney. Fear of Failure. New York: Van Nostrand: Reinhold, 1969.

EXERCISE—WHAT'S YOUR BLOCK TO CREATIVITY?

The following exercise can be used to reduce or eliminate a block to creativity. First, find some quiet time when you know you will not be disturbed or distracted. Take a pencil and paper and begin by labeling the paper " My Blocks to Creativity."

Start by writing down any thoughts that come to your mind as you think about your creative blocks. Let your thoughts flow without constraint. Write down everything that comes to you no matter its relationship to the topic. If you find this difficult, spend some time doodling on the paper when you feel blocked. Then look at the doodles and begin to associate your thoughts about blocks to the doodles. When you have written about a page or two, go back over it and underline in red pencil the significant statements you have made.

Look carefully at your underlinings. Turn these statements into clear, concrete statements about your blocks. For example — "I pay a lot of attention to what people think of me" might be restated more clearly as "I don't state my ideas about various problems because I feel they may not be accepted."

When you have turned your underlinings into clear statements of your blockages, put these statements on 3 x 5 index cards. Then put these cards somewhere in your immediate environment where you cannot fail to see them every day.

Everytime you believe you have behaved in a way that exhibits one of your blocks, make a mark on your index card. Be conscientious about keeping this record. Keep this tally for two weeks. At the end of this period add up the marks for each of your blocks.

Finally, take another tally of your blocks for a two week period. Compare this record with the previous two weeks. If you have been committed to changing your behavior you should notice a reduction in creativity blocking behavior. You may be on your way to unblocking your potential creativity.

EXERCISE — SHARING YOUR CREATIVE BLOCK

You need further help with your blocks when you have identified and carefully monitored them without this action leading to any behavior change.

Now is the time for peer consultation. Select a partner in your class or work group who is trustworthy and caring. Secondly, share the block to creativity with the partner. Collaboratively, come to a clear, concrete definition of the block. For example, "Every time I am in a group of five persons or more I never share my ideas." Or, "When I get halfway through a project I give up when I encounter a difficulty."

When the definition of the block is clearly stated, double check to see that it contains only *one* problem and that it is stated as specifically as possible.

Next, you and your partner each take a pad of paper and on each slip of the pad write one idea to resolve the block. Write as many ideas as you can in a five minute period. Then switch pads of paper and look through each other's ideas. If this triggers other ideas quickly write them down.

As a twosome, quickly rate each idea with either a plus or minus based upon its *feasibility* and *effect on the objective*. With your partner's help pick several ideas that form a strategy for overcoming your block. For example, if your block is related to lack of idea production in a group, you may decide to:

1. say one idea in a group each time you are a member of one;
2. announce to the group your problem so the group members can support your effort to produce ideas;
3. role play producing ideas in small groups, or
4. image a group with yourself producing ideas in it.

Contract with your partner to report on the results of your plan weekly. Identify results. If the plan does not work change it.

Chapter 4

Creative Problem Solving:
A Beginning

In Chapter 1, the Creative Problem-Solving model was introduced. Following its introduction I attempted to explain how creative problem-solving behavior was understood from various theoretical vantage points. Theories are used to guide the inventive practitioner's efforts in grappling with helping service problems. Following our foray into the theoretical forest, a number of barriers to creative action were identified. Awareness of such obstacles is a first step toward their resolution.

The goals of this chapter are to identify, more specifically, a number of guidelines useful in pursuing creative problem solving; to introduce several techniques that can be employed to gain sensitivity about issues in helping service practice; and to introduce the first stage of the CPS model: *fact-finding*.

CREATIVE GUIDELINES

It is important to understand a number of fundamental creative guidelines before learning to use the CPS model. The guidelines have been drawn from the three mainstreams of creativity theory. Although such guides, as I am presenting them, are abstract they can be actively applied if kept in the forefront of the problem-solver's thinking. With practice these guidelines become *internalized*, changing thinking intended to be creative to *creative thinking skill*.

Each creative guideline presented below is accompanied by a problem that illustrates the use of the guideline. Try to solve the problems, as your attempt at solution will clarify the guideline's meaning and value.

Generating Ideas

Problem 1—within a *five* minute time period write down all the ideas that are elicited by this question: what are the benefits to you, the helper, and to clients of *not* forming relationships with clients?

When the time is up count how many ideas you produced. Unless you have had the opportunity to put into practice the guideline this problem illustrates it's unlikely that you generated many ideas. Why not? Reflect upon what you were thinking as you attempted to produce ideas to this question. Did you think: "what could be good about *not* forming relationships with clients? How could we help a client without doing so? Why would someone think something good could come from something that hinders helping?" Such thoughts are frequent when we haven't practiced with the creative guideline of *deferred judgment*. This is the free production of ideas without evaluating them. Deferring judgment helps us think of ideas in several ways. First, we do not jump to conclusions, becoming fixated upon the first idea that comes to us. Secondly, by deferring judgment we allow ourselves time to generate many ideas; and so the evaluation of such a large quantity of ideas has a good chance of yielding high quality ideas (D'Zurilla & Nezu, 1980).

Past educational experiences have made it hard for us to defer judgment. We are taught to think critically, finding flaws in arguments or proposals. We draw upon logical thought that rules out ideas that do not follow a step-by-step or sequential flow. Ideas are judged, either because they are viewed as good or bad, or because the person presenting the idea may be negatively perceived.

Deferring judgment is not dissimilar to the helping service use of respect, or unconditional positive regard (Rogers, 1957). And when unconditional positive regard is ably used it produces results similar to deferred judgment. The client who knows that her helper is not judging her, produces thoughts, opinions and feelings more freely than a client who perceives that she is being evaluated. The helper who does not judge herself while generating ideas produces more of them than the helper who looks critically at those she produces.

Further, helping service students who understand and use deferred judgment are accepting of *unusual* ideas and willing to listen to them. Students who had taken my Creative Problem-Solving course showed significant changes in their willingness to entertain such ideas.

Finally, Guilford has suggested that deferred judgment is the condition that leads to *divergent thinking*, the kind of thought he has identified as producing creative ideas (1967). Divergent thinking is required in each stage of the CPS model.

Creative Guideline 1 — deferred judgment, or non-evaluative thinking — allows helping service workers and students to produce many ideas in the search for those that are creative.

Time Out

Problem 2 — below is a brief problem situation. Using the creative guideline of deferred judgment write all of your solutions to it until your thinking is *exhausted* of ideas.

> Lillian Adams has been married to her husband, John, for five years. Lately he has been moody, irritable, and often violent and abusive to her. Lillian is the mother of two boys, whose ages are five and three.

Now that you have become exhausted of ideas, involve yourself in another activity that has nothing to do with the problem. For example, take a walk around your neighborhood. Plan a meal for tomorrow. Or lie on the floor or bed and let your mind wander. Give yourself a "time out" of fifteen minutes.

Come back to the problem of Lillian Adams after the fifteen minute interlude is complete. Again, using the creative guideline of deferred judgment think of all the other ideas you now have to solve this problem.

Evaluate the ideas that your produced during both sessions by comparing the two lists. Are there any differences between the two sets of ideas produced? Did you produce more ideas during the first or second session? In your estimation, was there any difference in *quality* between the ideas you produced in the first idea-getting session as compared to the second? Did you receive a flash of insight or an "aha" when you were generating ideas after the break?

You have just practiced incubation as an approach for getting better ideas after becoming exhausted of solutions to a problem. Incubation can be defined as the practice of not consciously attending to a problem for a period of time (Guilford, 1979). Figure 10 demonstrates the incubation process graphically. The time given to incubation may vary with the problem under consideration and may involve minutes, hours, months or even years.

Does incubation always work? No, it doesn't. It works most frequently when we have worked on a problem for an extended time (Silveira, 1971). Why does it work? Sometimes we need to be refreshed physically and mentally. It may work because during the incubation period we discover other aspects of the problem. Or, when we have returned to the problem we may have gained a different perspective on it. Incubation is a behavior we practice naturally at times. But at other times we may try to *force* solutions to come without result. When we are stuck, a *time out* may facilitate creative problem solving.

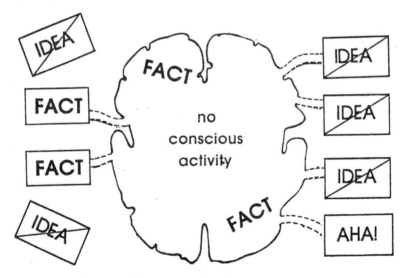

FIGURE 10. The incubation process.

Creative Guideline 2—incubation, particularly when we have worked on a problem for an extended period of time, may help produce better and/or more ideas for problem solution.

Breaking Out

Problem 3—connect all nine dots in the figure below with four straight lines without retracing any of your lines or lifting the pen from the page.

Your solution might look like this (see Figure 11).

As you can see the solution to the problem requires the problem solver to break the mental set suggested by the directions to the problem. These directions lead many problem solvers to understand the problem as one requiring that lines be joined within the boundaries constructed by the configuration of the dots. Figure 12 illustrates a typical incorrect solution based upon this assumption.

Staying within the parameters suggested by problem definitions can inhibit creative solutions. Breaking boundaries demands *two* separate creative acts. First, the problem solver must place an alternative meaning upon the way the problem is apparently defined.

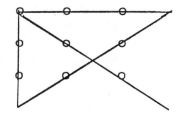

FIGURE 11. A correct solution to the nine dot problem.

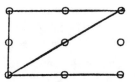

FIGURE 12. Incorrect solution to the nine dot problem.

Although the nine dot problem apparently suggests that the four lines should be drawn within the confines of the dots, in actuality the directions do *not* require such solutions. Secondly, after producing another problem perspective the problem solver then searches for a solution appropriate to this different perspective.

Can we relate this kind of problem to helping service practice? Let's consider this situation: a helper reads the assessment made by a helper previously involved with a disturbed child. Prior to meeting the child the helper reaches conclusions about the nature of the problem and how he must intervene to help the child. Although such early designations of problems are often made only by inexperienced or inflexible helpers it is clear that *all* helpers must approach helping situations with the capacity to look at them with fresh perceptions.

Creative Guideline 3—breaking out of mental sets is necessary for producing new problem definitions and solutions.

Discovery

Problem 4—how many squares do you see in Figure 13?

As you look at this figure you may first see that there are sixteen squares. Upon looking further you may see more squares. Note that all the smaller squares comprise one large square. The four squares on the top left, lower left, top right and lower right make up squares. Five squares in the center, center left, center right, center top and center bottom are also made up of four squares. Finally, a square can be made by cutting off four squares from the top and three from the right side. This action can yield three more squares by cutting four and three squares from a top, bottom, or side of the whole figure. Therefore, there is a total of $16 + 1 + 4 + 5 + 4 = 30$ (thirty) squares in the figure.

What we have done in discovering thirty squares in this figure is *to notice*. First we looked for squares, little ones, and then as we moved visually about the figure we began to notice patterns—that the smaller squares composed themselves into larger ones.

Noticing as a creative activity requires *relaxed attention*, a paradoxical state in which the problem solver is alert but not tense.

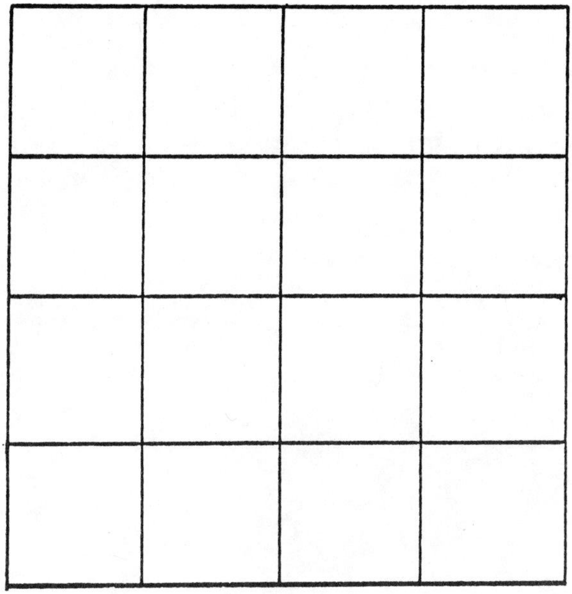

FIGURE 13.

There is a combination of a feeling of readiness and receptivity to stimuli. The noticer allows his attention to wander, hoping thereby to discover other possibilities. In noticing, then, we are open to opportunities that do not necessarily fit with any preconceived plan or idea.

Counsellors, social workers and psychotherapists use unfocused attention, or noticing, to understand the meta-language or the subtext of the communications they receive. Noticing is akin to what the great psychoanalyst Theodore Reik called "listening with the third ear" (1949).

Noticing is particularly useful in getting new ideas and in Chapter 7 we will make use of its contribution to problem solving by employing it to generate ideas.

Creative Guideline 4 — noticing, or unfocused attention to possibilities and opportunities, is an important skill for use in creative problem solving.

Transformation

Problem 5—what do you see as you look at Figure 14?

As you look at Figure 14 you may have perceived more than one figure. This exercise demonstrates a principle from Gestalt psychology. When we perceive something we have organized our percep-

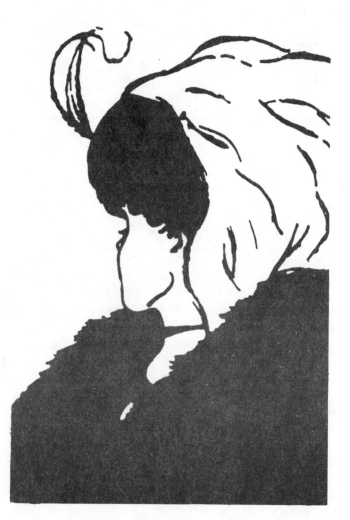

FIGURE 14.

tion into *figure and ground*. Objects that stand out from their context are readily seen. The background or the object's context is paid less attention. What such a principle suggests for creative behavior is that perception, i.e., what we register and make understandable, first by sensing and then through the imputation of meaning, can be rigid or flexible. The inability to flexibly move from figure to ground limits our perception of the world of phenomena. The counsellor knows, for example, that the goal of helping a maritally conflicted couple is ultimately to reduce the conflict. In the interim, the figure, i.e., the goal, must be forsaken for the ground, the immediate sub-goal of intensifying the conflict. Feelings and points of view long hidden (ground) surface, often causing anger and the intensification of conflict. Professional helpers know that the lay public views the solution of such conflict differently. That is, by suppressing the conflict it will go away. So we see that the helping service point of view regarding marital conflict and conflict in general is a *contrary recognition* or a reversal of figure and ground (Perkins, 1981).

Creative Guideline 5—flexibility of perception is produced by reversing figure and ground, and by perceiving things and ideas less dominant, when in parallel, than others. This helps define problems from a variety of perspectives and find novel solutions.

CREATIVE PROBLEM-SOLVING MODEL

CPS is a model and method that has been developed and used in solving problems in education, industry and the helping services. Issuing from the work of Alex Osborn (1963) and elaborated by Sidney Parnes (1977; 1981) the general CPS model emphasizes the alteration of divergent and convergent thinking throughout its stages. As Parnes describes the CPS training process and its goal:

> We try to help participants react first with imaginative play, then with tempered reality to a new fact, viewpoint, or idea. The open mindedness that we are seeking to instill relies upon how much imagination one first uses in approaching a thought before tempering it with reality. As a result . . . the participants can hopefully tolerate more ambiguity in a situation. In

the end, they can take more and more factors into consideration *in a given unit of time* while making decisions. (1977, p. 4)

How does CPS assist in helping service practice? First, by using creative guidelines within the CPS model and method helping service workers develop their ability to think fluently and flexibly (Klau & Gelfand, 1984). Being able to produce more and varied ideas should make the helper able to cope with problematic situations by: (1) better understanding them, and (2) seeing more alternatives for their solution. Fluent and flexible thought is a prerequisite for creative practice in all helping service domains. By *modeling* such thought and also by helping clients learn to think creatively workers can impart the attitudes and skills that are important for solving problems.

Second, use of CPS can be valuable for their production of *social invention*. As Conger defines it, social invention is the development of new procedures, programs and social policy for human services (1974). I have found that undergraduate social work students are able to use CPS as a model for developing prototypical inventions for social work (Gelfand, 1982 a,b). For example, two students interested in helping young children deal with anger combed the fairy tale and fable literature and identified situations indicative of the expression of angry emotions. Drawing these scenes onto a long scroll, three foot high, they then showed these scenes to children as stimuli for discussion of angry feelings. The children were able to identify with the situations and characters on the scroll and found they could then consider alternatives to inappropriate angry outbursts.

CPS can be joined with Thomas's Developmental Research and Utilization model for the purpose of social invention (Gelfand, 1982c). As CPS is a model that incorporates within it a creative methodology it can be a valuable tool for use in what Thomas calls the *generative process*, that process that demands the creative ideas be produced and elaborated for novel adoption, assembly and invention (Thomas, 1978).

Third, CPS can be used as an aid in social research. Use of its fact-finding and problem-finding stages can help researchers by expanding their knowledge base and so help them frame a number of different problems. The importance of formulating problems as a distinct and creative act has been identified by Einstein and Infeld (1938):

> The formulation of a problem is often more important than its solution, which may be merely a matter of mathematical or experimental skill. To raise new questions, new possibilities, to regard old problems from a new angle, requires imagination and marks real advance in science.

In sum, the value of the use of CPS as model and method, resides in its power to increase practitioners' ability to think fluently and thereby modeling such thinking skill for clients; for the use of defining and solving various helping service problems; for use as an aid in the invention of helping service procedures, programs and policy; and as a tool for assisting social researchers in knowledge development and problem formulation.

SENSITIVITY TO HELPING SERVICE CONCERNS

The inventive practitioner begins the CPS process when a *concern* is sensed. This sensitivity to concerns can be defined as the capacity to *become aware* of elements that indicate that something is wrong and the wrongness of something represents an opportunity. For example, a counselor in reviewing his caseload may notice that many of his clients, although seemingly well motivated and responsive to his interventions, remain stuck in their problem. The creative practitioner views this finding as both a *concern* and an *opportunity*. He asks "what is it about my clients that is blocking them from movement? What might I be doing to keep them from progressing?" As he collects data on his noticed concern the counsellor may frame a problem. Further, he may discover a new way to divert his clients from this counseling impasse. Like the man who finds he has a hole in his shoe, the counselor can opt to fix the shoe and then looks beyond this solution to ways of preventing holes from coming about.

What makes some helpers good at sensing concerns and opportunities while other helpers show little capacity to do so? I believe it is the ability *to notice* that differentiates these two groups. Noticing, remember, is the ability to engage in an unfocused search. It requires relaxed attention, whereby the searcher is willing to admit any kind of information into his understanding of problems or the generation of solutions to them. The noticer recognizes *patterns*, and often these patterns are transformed into issues and opportunities.

I asked a class of third and fourth year social work students to identify social work concerns they had noticed. These are a few:

— senior citizens and service delivery
— children and racism
— anger and children
— patients' rights
— student marriages
— social planning for communities
— stress in the helping professions

What makes these topics concerns and not problems? First, these topics are much too *broad* to be attacked as a problem. Secondly, the topics are *vague*. We may know little about them in a strictly factual sense, having drawn them as concerns because of personal involvement and observation. In order to view them as problems we must collect data about them and use the data in a selective way to frame problem statements and the problem questions about them.

Concerns are expressed in the beginning of the CPS process, then, are broad, vague topics little understood by their identifiers. They can be viewed as messes that require illumination by the collection of data and the formulation of problem statements and questions.

Learning to Sense Concerns and Opportunities

There are methods we can employ to help us become a better noticer of concerns. I want to introduce several of these methods for your use.

Key Words

One method of gaining sensitivity to concerns and opportunities is to use *key words* to stimulate our thinking. For example, let's take the word *aging* and associate it with the word *finances*. As you link these two words what possible concerns come to mind? I think of these: that many of the aged, I notice, are poverty-stricken; that the aged, in many instances, are on fixed incomes; that as I age I begin to worry more about my financial future; and that as the aged population grows, governments may have to expend greater resources to the social and health care of this grouping.

What I have done with these two words is force a relationship between them. As we do so, what appears at first glance to be two words without relevance to each other become associated and relevant.

Below is a two-column list of key words. Join pairs of words by choosing one from each column and then associating them. Identify possible concerns and issues as you link both words. Remember to consider *yourself* when you attempt to find concerns. Become sensitive to your own concerns as well as those that can be posed for others. Your concerns may easily be generalized to others.

Column A	Column B
school	love
friends	finances
family	racism
job	men personality
achievement	anxieties
neighbourhood	complications
career	organization
children	anger
disabled	leisure
religion	self-discipline
aging	belonging
house	creativity
sexuality	love
welfare	inefficiencies
relaxation	happiness

women   safety
poverty   body
marriage

(This exercise was adapted from Ruth Noller, Sidney J. Parnes and Angelo M. Biondi, *Creative Action Book* [New York: Charles Scribner's Sons, 1976], p. 6.)

The following are several examples of students' concerns generated by associating key words:

Karen: career ⟵――――――――――⟶ achievement

My chief concern about self-achievement would be that I have never really decided on or fall 'enough in love' with any one thing to seriously pursue it. Only recently have I started to allow myself to find social work interesting and worth commitment.

Bill: career ⟵――――――――――⟶ relationships

My concern is that there seems to be a conflict of interest between the time and energy I devote to my job and the time and energy I devote to a close relationship. The more time I spend on the job the better off I will be financially and I will be more secure. But will I have a feeling of belonging? What's more important to me?

Helen: neighbourhood ⟵――――――――⟶ anger

"I'm concerned about my neighbourhood. Angry, too. There are unemployed people in hotels and bars and on the streets day and night. There is danger of violence. I'm afraid to walk the streets. This isn't just a local problem."

As can be seen, the students, with the aid of the key words, got in touch with some issues of serious concern to them. The key word method may also be used to help clients identify thematic concerns for discussion.

The Question Checklist

Another good method for becoming more sensitive to concerns is to use a question checklist. Consider the set of questions below:

1. What is too complicated?
2. When is it best to listen?
3. How can you improve yourself?
4. With whom do you have problems getting along?
5. When do you believe you will be truly happy?
6. What is your goal in life?
7. What things are holding you back?
8. What makes social work hard for you?
9. In what ways are you inefficient?
10. What has angered you lately?
11. What would you really like to achieve in the next six months?
12. What would you like to change?
13. What excites you?
14. What ideas do you want to put in operation?
15. Of what are you most afraid?
16. What do you value most?
17. What is the most vulnerable part of your personality?
18. What angers you politically?
19. What must you do to feel financially secure?
20. In what ways would you like to help someone?
21. What groups in your community need support?

Responding freely to a question by writing down your thoughts about it may lead to the realization of a *significant concern*. For example, consider this question and this student's response to it:

Susan — How can I improve myself?

Basically I would like to be good to myself, to treat myself well and be in tune with myself. To be able to hear what I *really* am saying. To know what I want — so often what I say I want is tied up with what I know someone else wants or what they want me to want. I would like to be able to feel and express anger without the paralyzing fear of hurting others. I'd like to be able to use my power to the full. Right now I feel I have my feet on both the accelerator and the brake. I would like to like myself so solidly that it wouldn't matter to me whether I made a good impression on others or not. I would like to feel more satisfied with myself.

Susan has identified several concerns. She is concerned about her excessive need for approval and the effect it has upon expressing her genuine feelings. The question has raised concerns for her that she wishes to resolve.

Martha — What is the most vulnerable part of my personality?

Gentleness — empathy — sympathy. I find that in dealing with people I focus on their problems more than I do on my own needs and desires. Consequently in sympathy and in understanding their problem I attempt to help. This often happens with friends where I'm giving my time to fulfill their needs and I am left stranded.

Martha is identifying an important concern — meeting her needs without sacrificing or blunting the sensitivity that she has for others. She views her sensitivity as a negative personality quality because she has not yet learned to request from others something for herself.

The act of writing thoughts on paper helps to crystallize what may have begun as a vague feeling or a series of disconnected thoughts. Writing down thoughts requires a discipline that turns them into a form that helps us understand how thoughts and feelings are related.

(This exercise was adapted from Sidney J. Parnes, *The Magic of Your Mind* [Buffalo: Creative Education Foundation, Inc., 1981], p. 143.)

FACT-FINDING: THE FIRST STAGE OF CPS

Fact-finding is the data collection stage of CPS. It is the precursor to assessment. Perlman (1957), Bloom (1975), Reid and Epstein (1972), Compton and Galaway (1984) and Pincus and Minahan (1973) all identify a data collection stage as coming before the definition of the problem. Collecting and evaluating data is not a goal in itself. It is a means to the end of understanding the concern that has been noticed so we may *creatively* define the problem.

As can be seen in Figure 15 fact-finding is composed of two distinct phases, one requiring divergent, the other convergent thinking. The problem solver ideates and then evaluates her products.

What data does the inventive problem solver attempt to find? Because the first phase of fact-finding is a *divergent* phase the problem solver attempts to generate *any* question related to the concern. Employing the creative guideline of deferred judgment, the problem solver allows herself the freedom of posing questions without consideration of their importance, relevance or logical relation to the concern.

Fact-finding questions are produced by using a simple checklist of interrogatives — who? what? where? why? how? when? In generating questions we consider such categories as time, space, texture, shape, structure, function, magnitude and substance. For example, let's consider the concern of *community resources for abusive parents*. The following are some of the questions that can be generated using the checklist and some of the categories noted above:

> How can we find out what resources exist for abusive parents? (substance)
>
> Where do abusive parents go when they need help? (space)
>
> Who wants to provide resources for abusive parents? (function)

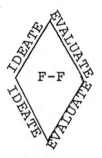

FIGURE 15. The fact-finding stage of CPS.

How do I feel about providing resources for abusive parents? (texture)

What abusive parents do I know?

What functions should community resources provide for abusive parents? (functions)

Why should abusive parents be provided community resources?

When do abusive parents need community services most? (time)

What does it feel like to be an abusive parent? (texture)

How large is the population of abusive parents? (magnitude)

When did abusive parents begin to be noticed? (time)

As can be seen, *any* question may be asked in the divergent phase of fact-finding. The limit to our question-asking is that of context and imagination. If we are seeing a client in a crisis situation our questions, both overt and covert, will be related to such factors as precipitating events, present coping strategies, and the client's present feeling state. If, however, we are part of a team working on the development of a new program to deliver crisis intervention services to newly widowed men and women, we in all likelihood, will have the luxury of using our imagination for generating many fact-finding questions without undue consideration to time.

Data begin to be gathered as the questions generated to the concern are answered through memory-produced information and consultation with experts, books, periodicals and other documents.

Upon completing our search for data we enter into the *second phase* of fact-finding by converging upon those facts that appear to be most useful and appropriate for transforming into problem statements and questions. This, of course, is an evaluative procedure requiring careful discrimination and judgment.

The difference between a normative problem-solving search for information and one instigated by a creative problem-solver is related to the divergent phase of the fact-finding stage. Because any question related to the concern is permitted, a potentially more valuable and comprehensive set of data may be compiled (Figure 16).

WORKING WITH SMALL CLIENT SYSTEMS

Reid has indicated that task-centered social work is a treatment modality with two goals: (1) that of helping the client solve an immediate problem, and (2) providing the client with a problem-solving strategy as a guide to the solution of any future problem (1978). In his task-centered approach clients are encouraged to generate possible solutions to the problems they face. Such behavior should help clients learn problem-solving skills that allow them to generalize to the various problems they will face in the future.

Fact-finding work can also proceed collaboratively. As a further step along the lines of helping clients learn problem-solving skills, practitioners, when working with individuals and marital pairs, might proceed by enlisting their aid in fact-finding work.

Frequently it is the practitioner who instigates a series of questions to which the client responds. This behaviour can be seen as modeling a problem-solving skill, that of question-asking. It would be better learned by clients if the worker followed this procedure:

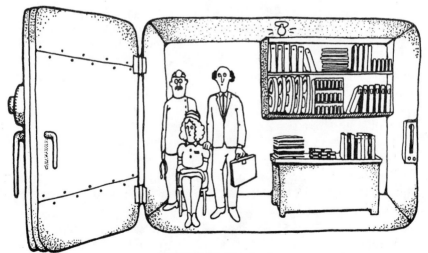

FIGURE 16. Data bank.

1. identify the purpose of question-asking (that of getting a clear understanding of the problem);
2. explain and teach deferred judgment to the client;
3. offer the client practice in question-asking; and
4. allow the client to pose any and as many questions as he wishes relating to his concerns.

Following this procedure, client and practitioner collaboratively attempt to get answers for all the questions posed and then select the information most important for understanding the client's concern and transforming it into a workable problem.

A situation similar to that in which clients are asked a number of questions about their concern is that of the classroom where teachers pose the questions and students function as respondents. It is crucial, however, that students learn how to form questions as they notice concerns. In so doing they learn an important problem-solving skill (Dillon, 1982). When clients and students use question-asking they become active participants in problem solving.

Summary

In this chapter I have introduced the beginning stage of the CPS model. Prior to its introduction I presented a set of guidelines for creative behavior. Discussed were *deferred judgment*, the practice of withholding judgment while searching widely; *incubation*, or the use of selective time outs for the purpose of eliciting fresh solutions; *noticing*, the practice of employing an unfocused search for uncovering patterns; *breaking boundaries*, or the attempt to break habitual or rigid thinking sets so problems and solutions can be perceived from an alternative perspective; and *reversal of figure and ground*, or the attempt to change what is seen to its opposite for a unique perspective.

The use of CPS begins with a sensitivity to concerns and opportunities and situations that indicate that something may be wrong or can be changed and possibly prevented.

Once a concern is sensed the first stage of CPS is begun by using fact-finding, thinking first divergently by posing questions, then by answering them and finally by converging upon selected data.

ADDITIONAL READINGS

Anne E. Fortune. "Problem-Solving Ability of Social Work Students," *Journal of Education for Social Work.* Vol. 20, No. 2, Spring, 1984, pp. 25-33.

Robert McKim. "Relaxed Attention" in *Guide to Creative Action.* Eds. Sidney J. Parnes et al. New York: Charles Scribner's Sons, 1977, pp. 206-211.

W.E. McMullan. "Creative Individuals: Paradoxical Personages," *Journal of Creative Behavior.* Vol. 10, No. 4, 1976, pp. 265-275.

Sidney J. Parnes and Angelo M. Biondi. "Creative Behavior: A Delicate Balance," *Journal of Creative Behavior.* Vol. 9, No. 3, 1975, pp. 149-157.

D.N. Perkins. *The Mind's Best Work.* Cambridge, Mass: Harvard University Press, 1981, pp. 78-83.

EXERCISE – FACT-FINDING 1

Using a concern or opportunity that you have identified by using the key words or checklisting technique, produce as many questions about the concern as you can within ten minutes. Begin the questions with who? what? where? how? why? and when? Then identify the questions that you can answer through memory produced information; those that can be answered by library research and those questions that can be answered by consulting experts.

EXERCISE – FACT-FINDING 2

Repeat the fact-finding 1 exercise in a group of 4 to 6 persons, using the same concern or opportunity you used in this previous exercise. Count your questions. Were you or the group more productive than when working as individuals?

As a group identify *how* each question can be answered. If time permits attempt to collect the data and then coverage upon the data considered relevant for defining problems.

EXERCISE – TWENTY QUESTIONS

One way to practice divergent thinking for fact-finding is to play Twenty Questions.

In this exercise two persons pair up. One person is designated the question-asker and the other is the person-with-the-problem.

The person-with-the-problem thinks about a problem that she needs to solve and identifies it without disclosing the problem to the question-asker.

The following guidelines can be helpful to the question-asker:

1 Begin by asking *any* question that you wish. Remember to start with the interrogative: who? what? where? why? how? when?
2. Ask as many open-ended questions as you can as they will help your person-with-the-problem to elaborate and give you much data. Ask close-ended questions to get necessary detail.
3. Listen attentively to the answers to the questions. they may give you clues as to the direction your question asking should go.

Attempt, as you get the answers to your questions, to put the information together. What kind of problem does it indicate? Attempt a specific answer. Find the problem by collecting as much data as twenty questions will allow.

Chapter 5

The Importance
of Finding the Problem

Problem finding is the creative problem-solving skill of formulating problem definitions from the data collected in the fact-finding stage. Problem finding in CPS is analogous to the assessment stage in various helping service problem-solving models (cf. Reid & Epstein, 1977; Compton & Galaway, 1984; Bloom, 1975; Perlman, 1957; Northen, 1981) (Figure 17).

Getzels (1975) has suggested the value of a conceptual distinction between *discovered problem situations* and *presented problem situations*. Problem situations can be meaningfully distinguished in terms of how much of the problem is clearly given at the start, how much of the method for reaching a solution is presently at hand, and how complete the agreement is as to what makes a good solution.

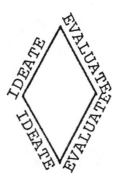

FIGURE 17. The problem-finding stage of CPS.

Helping service situations can be placed upon the continuum suggested by Getzels. At one end of this continuum are situations in which the problem, method, and the solution are already known. For example, a woman who is the single-parent head of a family of four children applies for welfare assistance. She hasn't any job skills, nor has she any past employment record. She has no visible means of support. Having this data the intake worker recognizes the importance of helping this family receive immediate assistance and then helping the mother become eligible for AFDC. In this situation the worker recognizes the problem easily, knows the method for application and applies it as the problem solution.

At the other end of the continuum are *discovered* problems, i.e., situations where the problem itself is yet to be formulated, must be identified and where the appropriate method for finding a solution and the nature of the solution is not yet known. Consider this example from the recent past. Until the mid-1950s there did not exist a theory to understand family problems or the family as a unit for helping intervention. Not until the ground-breaking work of Bateson, Jackson, Haley and Weakland (1956), Satir (1967) and Ackerman et al. (1961) did helping service workers view family interactions as problematic; interest themselves in developing treatment methods for dysfunctional families; and in applying a systems approach for treatment. In another famous example of problem discovery, Freud, through his interest in the neurotic, found that their symptoms could be understood and this understanding, coupled with the invention of psychoanalysis, led to a reduction of their disabling symptoms. Freud's creativity originated in his concern for discovery, his ability to approach a situation in which there was a problem yet to be discovered, i.e., how to understand the neurotic; to find that problem; to invent a method for reaching a solution; and, to an extent, solving it.

USING PROBLEM-FINDING METHOD
IN HELPING SERVICE PRACTICE

Clearly, most helping service situations tend to fall on that part of the problem-finding continuum where there is some degree of problem understanding at the start, where much of the method for reaching a solution is readily available and where there is some agreement about what constitutes a good solution. In what ways then can problem-finding, as a problem-solving skill, be used creatively for helping service practice?

Creative problem-finding can offer the direct practice worker a way to develop multiple perspectives on the social situation of the client system. Normative problem-solving models frequently call for a problem definition; creative problem-solving asks that the problem-solver *diverge* so that many definitions may be generated. The expectation is that the generation of many differing problem perspectives will lead to one or several that allow for a fluent and flexible application of solutions. For if the problem definition is good, i.e., creative, it frees both helper and client to think of and imagine many quality solutions to the problem. A poor assessment of the problem does the reverse; it restricts our ability to produce good alternatives for solution. In studying the effects of problem definition upon the generation of alternatives, Nezu and D'Zurilla (1981b) found that training individuals in problem definition techniques increased the quality of solutions to socially oriented test problems. Although these authors' methods for problem definition are but partially identical to those used in CPS, such results suggest the *importance* of problem-finding for generating good problem solutions.

Problem-finding is not only a valuable problem-solving skill for the direct practice worker, it also can be employed effectively by the helping service researcher. The ability to frame hypotheses fluently and flexibly can lead to new ways of viewing old helping service research problems, thereby opening up new lines of inquiry. The planner and administrator can use creative problem-finding to develop new goals and objectives for service programs. Further, because producing good problem definitions increases the likelihood of generating good solutions, problem-finding should be considered an important skill in the development of new helping service technology. It should then find use in Rothman's Social R&D model (1981) and Thomas's Developmental Research and Utilization Schema (1978). Problem-finding, then, can be an important problem-solving skill for the invention of procedures, programs and policy for helping service professionals (Gelfand, 1982c).

CREATIVE PROBLEM-FINDING: EXAMPLES

Direct Practice

Problem definition can be one of the most creative acts of helping service practice. For example, let's observe a helping service worker attempting to establish a relationship with a neglecting parent. The worker has some data about the social situation. She knows that the client has had an extremely poor relationship with her own mother, who was alcoholic and abusive to her. She was deprived, herself, of physical and emotional nurturance. The client, the helping service worker knows, feels inadequate as a mother and becomes quite hostile when the worker attempts to help her. These facts lead the worker to initially assess the client problem as related to a hostile-dependent attitude, leading the client to resist help because of her fear of becoming involved with, dependent upon, and subsequently rejected by the worker. The worker then attempts to intervene based upon the guidance provided by this problem assessment.

By employing deferred judgment the creative problem-solver views the above hypothesis as only one of a range of hypotheses that can be made based upon the data. The following definitions are alternatives that could be used as guides to helping service work intervention:

1. The client may not be hostile-dependent. This is *my* label, and behavior I expect based upon my training. *How can I modify my expectations of the client?*
2. The client is inadequate as a mother but apparently is adequate in other areas of social living. *How can I find ways of using these areas of adequacy to improve our relationship?*
3. Rather than being hostile-dependent toward me, the mother is hostile-dependent toward those I represent. *How can I find ways of separating myself from those I represent?*
4. The client is not afraid of becoming involved with me; she is afraid of her hostility and dependency. *How can I minimize her hostile-dependent fears by maintaining a minimal level of involvement?*

5. The mother may be hostile to me, but I, also, may be hostile to her. *How can I reduce my hostile reactions toward her?*
6. The mother is resistant to me and I am perceiving that as a negative element. *How can I make use of the mother's resistance to me so I can develop a good relationship with her?*

The immediate assessment of the client's difficulty and reactions toward the worker requires specific interventions based upon the client's hostile-dependent attitude. Unless this assessment leads to creative problem solutions, however, it will be ineffective. By looking at the known facts about the client, and by viewing them in differing perspectives the worker is able to produce a number of different hypotheses, each of which, may lead to fruitful, and flexible solutions. *The major yardstick for an assessment's effectiveness is the opportunity it presents its user for producing good solutions.*

Kadushin (1963) has written that helpers frequently develop client assessments that can be identified as descriptions of their "Aunt Fanny." What Kadushin has in mind are those assessment statements that could relate to *anyone's* Aunt Fanny. For example:

The client has difficulty in performing at optimal capacity when under stress.

The client has unresolved dependency feelings.

The client has unconscious hostile urges.

Kadushin responds to these cliché statements—"so has your Aunt Fanny."

To determine whether social workers might be susceptible to such valueless generalities he designed a study in which MSW supervisors rated the validity of what they thought were second year graduate social work students' diagnostic summaries. Each of three groups of supervisors were given a different case summary but identical assessments to the different case summaries. Thus, although each group read a different summary the assessment they were to rate, upon reading these summaries,were identical for each group. All three groups of supervisors rated the *fake* student assessments as slightly above average, indicating that the different assessments had nearly equal validity for the supervisors involved in this study. Frequently then assessments may be of little value in differentiating and individualizing clients. The ability to generate many different assessments may increase the probability of producing one or several that lead to a unique understanding of the client.

Social Policy

Another example of how problem-finding may be used is related to the area of social policy. The concern that is addressed is that of client rights in institutional settings. The following are some of the facts used in finding problems within this social issue:

1. Client rights can be conceived as an issue of *legal* and, as well, *moral* nature. Individuals as citizens have rights defined by law. A moral view would consider the social welfare of the individual.
2. Recognition of client rights may be impeded by such factors as (a) agency mandate, e.g., worker's activities in this area may be blocked because of the legal boundaries of the agency; (b) the physical, emotional and mental abilities of the client – in this case a client may be unable to communicate to the worker that his/her rights are being violated; (c) the workers' attitude may be such that clients' rights are not considered; (d) societal constraints, such as exist in establishing group homes for the retarded and adolescent, may prevent rights of clients from being met; (e) rights may be violated because the client has not the financial resources to choose to live privately. (Consider the mental patient who may have no right to privacy at all, living on a ward with forty other patients.)
3. Clients may have recourse to private lawyers, human rights commissions and social workers who may advocate for them.

Using this data the problem finder formulates the problem in the following ways:

1. How can I enable clients to overcome various physical, mental and emotional blocks in exercising their rights?
2. How can I balance the tendency toward paternalism toward

clients with the need for advocacy in the area of client's rights?

3. How can I encourage clients to recognize and exercise their own rights in institutionalized settings?
4. How can I develop and implement tools which might be adapted to a variety of institutional settings for insuring client's rights?
5. How can I specifically define the issue of client's rights?
6. How can I encourage the social work profession's commitment to all client's rights?
7. How can I help change the mandate of those agencies that are inadvertently violating client's rights?
8. How can I help individual social workers become more aware of the issue of client's rights?
9. How can I expand the public's awareness of client's rights?
10. How can I coordinate the services of all professionals involved with the concern of client's rights?

The problem finder has produced ten problem statements that relate to the client rights concern. The number of statements generated is limited only by the problem finder's ability to think fluently and flexibly given the data at hand. From such problem-generating activity may come a unique perspective on the social policy issue under consideration.

PROBLEM-FINDING METHODS

There are a number of guidelines that can be employed to help us problem find creatively.

Guideline #1 — from the data collected in the fact-finding stage is produced one problem statement. It is begun with the phrase "How can I/we. . . ." This phrase is used because it suggests that to solve the problem various alternatives for solution must be considered.

For example: consider the client who is constantly depressed. He states: *How can I stop being depressed*?

Guideline #2 — finding the objective that lays underneath the problem as stated above will help us produce another problem statement. To do this we ask the question, "why do I want to stop my depression?'' The answer to the question leads us to a redefinition of the problem (Figure 18).

For example: Why do I want to stop my depression: "So I can enjoy my life" comes the answer. Therefore a new problem statement can be generated "how can I enjoy my life?"

The value of this restatement is that the problem statement has now moved to a higher level of abstraction. By so doing the depressed person can now consider the various domains of total life functioning for providing possible enjoyment rather than focus upon a circumscribed illness. There is now the opportunity of finding many more ways of enjoying oneself than of finding techniques to treat a depression.

Guideline #3 — another way to restate problems is to change the structure of the problem statements. By modifying various sentence parts or by using different verbs new problem perspectives can be gained.

For example: "how can I enjoy life?" can be changed to "how can I learn those activities that make me feel good?" or "how can I develop interests that stimulate and excite me?" (Figure 19). Such problem formulating may help the problem finder to discover a definition that best lends itself to finding creative solutions to it.

Guideline #4 — by asking why? we are able to find the objective we are striving for in our problem statement. There is another question that can be posed that helps in restating problems. That question is "what's stopping me?" By so doing, an answer can be re-

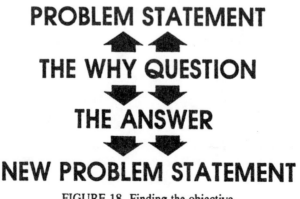

FIGURE 18. Finding the objective.

ceived that is specific and leads to a problem statement that suggests finding concrete solutions (Figure 20).

For example: "how can I develop interests that stimulate and excite me?" What's stopping me? "I don't know what they are" comes the answer. Using this answer a new problem statement—"how can I *find* these activities that stimulate and excite me?"—is formed. The what's stopping me question helps the problem finder to get a narrowly defined problem statement; one that suggests to the finder specific solutions to it.

Guideline #5—when a large quantity of problem definitions are produced and the practitioner is satisfied with this work, a selection among the definitions must be made. As in all good problem-solving methods, if the problem definition chosen is broad it must be partialized (Figure 21). Breaking the broad problem definition into sub-problems makes the overall work demanded for solving the problem appear less onerous and allows for a step-by-step approach to its mastery.

A STUDENT PROBLEM-FINDS

The example of student problem-finding that follows demonstrates the basic strategy for problem-finding.

The student's concern is racism and its effect on youth in society.

How can I learn those activities that make me feel good?

How can I develop interests that stimulate and excite me?

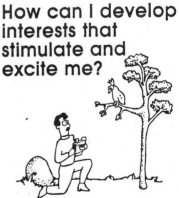

FIGURE 19. Changing the parts of sentences.

PROBLEM STATEMENT
THE WHAT'S STOPPING ME QUESTION
THE ANSWER
NEW PROBLEM STATEMENT

FIGURE 20. Using the "What's stopping me" question.

She converges in the following *facts* elicited from the fact-finding stage:

1. racial attitudes are learned,
2. racial attitudes of children can be positively shaped,
3. positive racial attitudes can prevent racism,
4. socialization techniques can be employed with various societal groupings to enhance understanding and understanding of racial groups,
5. helping service workers can be trained to carry out these socialization tasks,
6. new techniques must be developed to help children affected by racism,
7. techniques can be used at the macro or societal level to prevent racism.

Problem Definitions

Why do I want to do this? (What's stopping me?)

1. How can I make children more aware, understanding and accepting of all racial groups?

2. How can I develop a plan of action comprised of various socialization techniques for the *purpose of preventing racism from occurring at all levels of society*?

3. How can I change public attitudes?

4. How can I stimulate *public concern* over racism?

5. How can I organize the public to take concrete steps to alleviate racism?

6. How can I organize a task force for the purpose of fostering racial awareness in society?

(What's stopping me?)

7. How can I encourage influential public institutions, such as schools, religious organizations and community centers to work toward erasing racism?

8. How can I *enable helping service practitioners* to better help young victims of racism to work on their feelings of racial inferiority and negative self-concepts?

9. How can I *stimulate helping service researchers* to delve deeper into the problems of racism and its effect on youth, so that new treatment modes can be developed?

10. How can I *make parents and teachers aware* of the necessity of promoting positive racial attitudes and high self-esteem in children?

11. How can I encourage teachers to enhance positive racial identities in a multi-racial setting?

12. How can I organize parent self-help groups for the purpose of motivating other parents in this area of concern?

13. How can I motivate concerned children to organize self-help groups in order to fight racism amongst their peers?

In problem definition #2 the student formulates a problem with the recognition that racism can encompass all of society. However, the task she has been given is to invent social technology to deal with racism in the immediate future. Because of this she selects problem definition #8 as that more readily workable for solution given the immediacy of this time frame.

A PROBLEM-FINDING MODEL

Dillon (1983) has formulated a model of problem-finding involving two basic dimensions. He identifies the *existential* and *psychological* dimensions of problem-finding. By existential Dillon means the determination of a problem's status in the world of events. Problems, he says, can be either *existent*, *emergent*, or *potential*. An existent problem is one that has fully developed being and appearance. The psychological relationship between problem and observer in the case of an existent problem is that the problem is evident, i.e., recognizable. Emergent problems, a second, less developed level, suggests a problem that is implicit. The observer, on a psychological level, after probing the data *finds* the problem. The most difficult problem-finding level in Dillon's scheme considers problems as existentially *potential*. No problem exists as a phenomena in the real world; the observer finds apparently irrelevant or non-related elements and creates a synthesis — a new problem. Figure 22 identifies the existential and psychological dimensions of each problem-finding level and the corresponding activity required of the problem finder.

I want to suggest a way in which Dillon's model of problem-finding can be related to helping service activities. The *levels* of problem helpers are involved with are related to the helper's *function*, his *workplace*, and the *population* that is served. For example, consider the helping service planner who is employed on a govern-

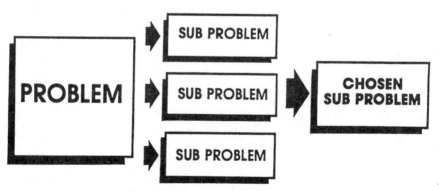

FIGURE 21. Partializing the problem.

	Existential	Psychological	Activity
Level 1	existent	evident	recognition
Level 2	emergent	implicit	discovery
Level 3	potential	not noticeable	invention

FIGURE 22. Dillon's model of problem finding.

mental level and is involved in planning mental health services with a team comprised of mental health professionals. Hypothetically, this planner should be involved in the collection and analysis of community data prior to any definition of problem. The assumptions that I make in this situation are: (1) that the social planner, as part of a team of professionals, must share data collaboratively before any problem finding is undertaken, and (2) even though mental health problems may be apparent, the population targeted for service is too complex to be understood without thorough analysis. Therefore, the social planner's problem-finding efforts should fall in Level 2 of Dillon's framework.

Let's take another example. Consider the front line helper investigating child abuse from a child welfare setting. Frequently, the helper is given a problem as identified by the community. Data have been collected on the alleged abusing parents by teachers, doctors, nurses, neighbors, relatives and other community representatives. The helper, without much further investigation, *knows* a problem exists (Level 1). But there is another problem that the helper must find. The worker must assess the family situation, its strengths, weaknesses, potential for change, resources, etc., so that a treatment plan can be made. Because the data necessary to find this problem are only gained through ongoing collaboration with the family unit and require frequent hypothesis formulation and reformulation, the worker is engaged in problem-finding on the second level of Dillon's model.

Here is one final example of how we can relate Dillon's problem-finding schema to helping service activities. A helping service agency has mandated a group of external researcher-planners to develop a new form of service delivery to young families at risk. The agency has collected some data on this clientele and believes that young families are highly vulnerable to high levels of stress and disorganization. Although agency administrators and helpers have some ideas about the form that the new service should take, the agency has agreed to allow the external group complete freedom in coming forth with their proposals.

The group begins its work by collecting data, some already generated by the agency and other data the group believes they need to understand the problem. The researcher-planners then produce a host of problem definitions related to the at-risk group. They finally select a problem definition that points toward a primary prevention program for young families in the community.

The example indicates that the research team was problem-finding on Dillon's Level 2. Existentially, there is an emergent status to the situation, a situation in which the group must discover a problem implicit within it. We cannot rule out that there may be elements of Level 3 problem-finding involved in this situation. The data when actively probed may not yield discovery of a problem. The data may be contradictory, apparently impossible to reconcile, and appear as non-relevant. Hence, the research group may enter into problem-finding Level 3, where they are involved in creatively synthesizing apparently irreconcilable data toward the act of *inventing* a problem.

Summary

Problem-finding refers to the active search for creative definitions that are formed from the data compiled in the fact-finding stage of CPS. As we have seen problem-finding proceeds from a simple act on one end of the continuum where the problem finder is given the problem, knows the method of solution and knows what the appropriate solution should be. On the other parts of the continuum are problems that require discovery and invention, whereby the method to solve them is relatively unknown and there is little or no agreement as to the appropriate solution.

Problem-finding, as a stage in the CPS process, can be facilitated through a specifiable methodology. The problem finder must first produce a problem statement from the data collected in the fact-finding stage. Using such techniques as asking "why? and what's stopping me?" and restructuring problem definitions helps the problem finder generate many problem-finding statements. Therefore, problem-finding initially involves a divergent search for problems; following this search the problem finder converges on the most fruitful problem definition, i.e., the one that promises to elicit creative ideas to the problem.

Dillon's problem-finding scheme has been discussed and I have attempted to relate it to the problem-finding work frequently done in the helping services. Do the helping services ever problem-find on what Dillon calls the *potential* level of problem-finding, that of the activity of inventing problems? Seldom, seems to be the answer. Because the helping services are professions in which most workers are faced with demanding and serious problems that frequently require immediate relief, workers seldom have the luxury of the long divergent search that inventing problems requires. Perhaps the interest that Thomas (1978) and Rothman (1981) are generating with their new developmental research methodologies will encourage researchers and planners to *invent* problems for the helping services.

ADDITIONAL READINGS

A. Nezu and T. J. D'Zurilla. "Effects of Problem Definition and Formulation on Decision-Making in the Social Problem-Solving Process." *Behavior Therapy*, Vol. 12, 1981, pp. 100-106.

M. Csikszentmihalyi and J. W. Getzels. "Discovery-Oriented Behavior and the Originality of Creative Products: a Study with Artists." *Journal of Personality and Social Psychology*, Vol. 19, No. 1, 1971, pp. 47-52.

J. W. Getzels. "The Problem of the Problem." In Hogarth, P. M. (Ed.), *Question Framing and Response Consistency*. San Francisco: Jossey-Bass, 1982.

R. S. Crutchfield. "Nurturing the Cognitive Skills of Productive Thinking." In *Life Skills in School and Society*, Washington, D.C.: Association for Supervision and Curriculum Development, 1969.

J. T. Dillon. The Multidisciplinary Study of Questioning. *Journal of Educational Psychology*, Vol 754, 1982, pp. 147-165.

J. Smilansky. "Problem Solving and the Quality of Invention: an Empirical Investigation." *Journal of Educational Psychology*, Vol. 76, No. 3, pp. 377-386.

PROBLEM-FINDING EXERCISE

When you find a problem, is it the problem you really want? The test of whether a problem is really a problem is to get underneath it to see if it really has an objective. The following helping service problems require you to ask of them "why do I want to do this?" Once you have the answer (if there is one) use it to produce another problem statement.

Problem 1

Ralph Hughes, a social work supervisor in a local public assistance agency, found that one of his workers was constantly late for work. Further, although this worker was adequate in his work with clients she also handed in reports, time sheets and other paper work after Ralph's specified deadlines. Ralph conceptualized the problem this way — "how can I get rid of this worker who is causing me so much difficulty?"

Your Problem Statement:_____

_____

_____

Problem 2

A large family service agency found that its family workers were turning over their cases very rapidly. Cases, whether individual, marital or family units were being seen on the average of four visits. There was little variation of this average among workers. Administration, believing this data suggested that clientele were not being "held" adequately for proper help to be given, framed the problem statement this way:

"How can we help workers increase the average number of times they see clients?

Your Problem Statement:_____
_____
_____

Problem 3

Ruth Williams, a helping service student who is placed in a neighbourhood enters work with a group of unwed mothers. Her field consultant meets with her and her placement supervisor to determine her progress. In the meeting Ruth answers her supervisors and field consultant's questions curtly and abruptly. She does not explain her work in depth and appears to be angry about having to justify her actions with her group. After the meeting the field consultant states the problem as "How can I help Ruth relax in these progress meetings?"

Your Problem Statement:_____
_____
_____

Problem 4

A client, Ron Alwin, comes to individual counseling every week. Seen by his counselor for the last two months as cooperative, motivated and energetic, nevertheless, the counselor had to admit to herself that Ron was not really changing. Mostly he talked openly and freely about himself and his stated problem of being afraid of intimacy. Counselor and client had explored this problem endlessly and it was decide by the counselor to restate the problem she was having with helping Ron move as "How can I help Ron talk about other topics in his life that might shed more light on his problem?"

Your Problem Statement:_____
_____
_____

PROBLEM-FINDING EXERCISE 2 – WHAT'S STOPPING YOU?

Problem-Finding in Pairs

Pair up with a partner. Share some information about a situation you presently are not too clear about with your partner. From this information your partner will define your problem. Following this your partner will ask you "what's stopping you?" You will give him the answer and from this answer your partner will restate your problem. Repeat this step in the exercise at least four times or until your partner feels comfortable in restating the problem from your answer to the "what's stopping you?" question. Following this part of the exercise your partner will now, starting with the last restatement of the problem, ask the question "why do you want to do this?" Repeat this question asking and restatement process until your partner can comfortably generate problem definitions from your answers.

Now reverse roles. Your partner should now share some information about *his* concern that is perceived as vague or unclear. Using both questions as techniques for problem finding, restate problems as your partner did with you. Practice until you develop competence in using these techniques.

EXERCISE – PROBLEM-FINDING FROM FACT FINDING

Below are a number of facts collected from a fact-finding stage of CPS. From these facts produce as many problem definitions as you can within a ten minute period.

- X wants to be a helping service consultant
- X is 29 years old
- she is skillful at mediating and making people feel comfortable, both individually and in groups
- X has never had to market herself

- X perceives professions and businesses outside of the helping services as more "tough-minded" than the helping services
- X wants to consult in family and marital therapy situations
- she has a masters degree in social work and three years of post-masters training in family therapy
- X has a good network of social work colleagues.

Write your problem definitions below:

1. _____
2. _____
3. _____
4. _____
5. _____
6. _____
7. _____
8. _____
9. _____
10. _____
11. _____
12. _____
13. _____
14. _____
15. _____
16. _____
17. _____
18. _____
19. _____
20. _____

EXERCISE – PARTIALIZING THE PROBLEM

Problem definitions may be selected because of their creative potential and yet be too broadly framed for effective problem-solving. Below is an example of using this skill.

Problem Definition – How Might I Help Ralph Develop His Identity?

1. *How might I help Ralph* identify the skills he believes he has?
2. *How might I encourage Ralph to explore his strengths and weaknesses*?
3. *How might I show Ralph how to explore his family heritage so he may connect with it*?

The key, in part, to partializing a broad problem definition is to redefine, in greater specificity, the major concepts of the broad definition. In problem definition 1 a major concept is the *development of identity*. This definition can then be partialized by conceiving of different and specific ways this development can be carried through. The question I ask and attempt to answer in doing so is this: of what is identity made? My answer – skills, strengths and weaknesses, and family heritage – help me to more concretely frame problems that are in workable form for problem solving. Below are a number of problem definitions that are broadly conceived. Break them down into their specifiable components.

Problem Definition – How Might I Develop a Physical Fitness Program for Senior Citizens?

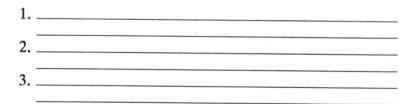

1. _____
   _____
2. _____
   _____
3. _____
   _____

Problem Definition—How Might I Organize my Neighbourhood to Take Action Against Vandalism?

1. _____
   _____
2. _____
   _____
3. _____

Problem Definition—How Might I Help the A Family to Reinforce Its Boundaries?

1. _____
   _____
2. _____
   _____
3. _____
   _____

Problem Definition—How Might I Encourage Mr. Alton to Find Work?

1. _____
   _____
2. _____
   _____
3. _____
   _____

Chapter 6

Strategy and Idea Finding:
An Introduction

Getting ideas should be easier if we have been effective in selecting a *good* problem definition. Einstein and Inhelder have said that a problem is frequently solved by good problem-finding work; the solution to it may only be the application of technical competence (1938).

However, we mustn't treat the ability to produce ideas cavalierly. Generating good ideas, fluently and flexibly, is a creative problem-solving skill that often requires much practice to acquire. Why is this so? In Chapter 2, remember, I mentioned our culture's narrow conception of intelligence. Essentially our schools are interested in teaching and rewarding a conceptual-logical intelligence. What this suggests is that thinking characterized by a *critical attitude* is reinforced during most of our learning lives in school. A critical attitude is that attitude characterized by skepticism, by a reluctance to believe. It stops us from jumping to conclusions without sufficient evidence. Characterized by logic and analysis it is an attitude that helps us to compare and contrast one experience with another, testing the present with the prior.

Critical thinkers, imbued with the critical attitude, see flaws in theory, attend to the logical flow of thought and show strength in carefully identifying why ideas may not work. Critical thinking is an important skill in CPS, particularly in the convergent phases of each stage (Figure 23).

Anderson has pointed out that the *creative attitude* is based upon the love of adventure more than the desire for certainty. It is an

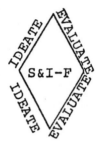

FIGURE 23. The strategy and idea-finding stage of CPS.

attitude that is forward looking in that it considers possibilities rather than what has gone before (1980, p. 66). The creative attitude, as we have seen, is described in theory by Barron and Rogers, is composed of an openness to experience and an internal locus of evaluation. The creative attitude tolerates ambiguities, doubts, and is not fearful of the unknown. There exists a freedom to explore, to be oneself and to express that which is within the individual without fear of censure and concern with evaluation (Stein, 1974, p. 24). It is the creative attitude that is used in producing ideas.

DEFERRAL OF JUDGMENT REVISITED

Chapter 4 introduced a number of guidelines that are considered important for creative problem-solving behavior. It is the ability to search broadly without invoking critical evaluation or judgment, and is the major factor in learning how to produce creative ideas. Because our culture so strongly emphasizes the critical component of thinking, it is necessary to ask ourselves and others to adopt an attitude of deferred judgment when generating ideas (Figure 24).

Of course, it would be fine if all we had to do was intellectually understand the idea of deferred judgment and then apply it. However, we must practice long and hard before the attitude is internalized. People of all ages and all backgrounds experience difficulty in applying it. For example, a student of mine said to me when I asked the class to practice it, "But what if you know the ideas people are thinking up are stupid or just won't work, why bother doing it?"

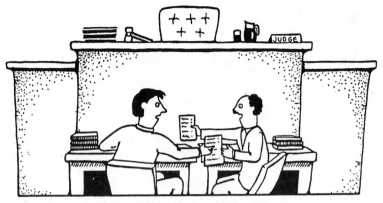

FIGURE 24. Deferred judgment.

The notion that an idea must be a common sense idea or one that is at the forefront of our thought, i.e., easily recalled, or that an idea must sound conventional or appropriate, is strongly ingrained in our thinking patterns.

Stating the deferred judgment guideline and simply asking individuals to follow it will not work. We need to put this guideline into practice, receive feedback on our performance and then with the understanding this feedback affords us practice more for additional competence.

But how do we practice deferring judgment? We require a technique that will help us learn deferred judgment and how to generate ideas at the same time.

BRAINSTORMING — AN IDEA-FINDING TECHNIQUE

Brainstorming is an idea-finding technique attributed to Alex Osborn (cf. Stein, 1975, p. 25). It is a group technique that emphasizes two major principles and four major rules. The two principles are *deferment of judgment* and *quantity breeds quality*. The four major rules are as follows:

1. criticism of self and others is ruled out;
2. that freewheeling is welcomed;
3. quantity of ideas is wanted; and
4. combination and improvement of ideas are sought.

Osborn thought that the judicial mind stopped the flow of creative ideas — therefore the principle of deferred judgment. The principle of quantity breeds quality is suggested by the way we frequently associate to a problem. First come ideas we easily remember, followed later by ideas less common or usual. To get to original ideas we must go through these conventional ideas and to do so we must produce many ideas. The rules come from the two basic principles. In order to defer judgment the brainstormer must not criticize his or her group member's ideas. Freewheeling encourages an idea to be considered, thereby relaxing the mind's censor and to think without significant inhibitions. Quantity is wanted because quality is wished; we hope in this way for original ideas. Finally by combining and improving upon the ideas already offered we encourage additional ideas and also exercise the right to modify ideas already put forward.

In the classic brainstorming session a specific problem is presented to the group. The group then produces as many ideas to the problem as it can within a specified time period. Group size is important to the functioning of a brainstorming group. Groups composed of 8 to 10 members appear to be ideal for the brainstorming task; smaller groups suffer from less input and therefore the generation of fewer ideas. Problems presented to a group must be clearly stated so that the group's ideas can relate effectively to the problem. Groups may record its own ideas by designating a member to do so but it is best to have an external recorder so all members of the group may be free to participate.

A facilitator is required when a group is learning to brainstorm. Because a good group process is crucial it is important that the facilitator observe this process and offer appropriate comments upon it. What kind of group dynamics occur during a brainstorming session? I have found that although group members may not criticize each other's ideas verbally, they may do so non-verbally. It is important to encourage congruence in the group member's behavior. It is also very important to observe the participation pattern of the brainstorming group. Are there too many ideas coming from too few members? Are patterns of dominance and powerlessness developing? It is essential for group members to participate as nearly equally as possible. If members, because of previous group experiences, put themselves in a non-participative position it is the facilitator's role to observe this and to comment upon it. The facilitator can also serve as a model and encourager. When the group becomes stuck the facilitator may contribute an idea, stimulating the group in this way. Exhorting the group to think of further ideas frequently helps because members may hold back ideas early in their learning of brainstorming for fear of appearing silly — or too unconventional.

However, the facilitator must not stand in the way of group members' enjoyment of the brainstorming process. For, if the group learns to adhere to the brainstorming principles and rules it *will* have fun. As the group becomes less inhibited and less bound by the restrictions of normal group behavior, its ideas will become more unusual, funny and absurd. And some of them will spark spontaneous hilarity. Guidelines for evaluating a good brainstorming session are the amount of good humor generated by it, as well as its capacity for producing good ideas.

Learning Brainstorming — Exercising Deferred Judgment

It's important that you be in to learn how to defer judgment before we progress to other idea-finding techniques. If you have done the exercises at the end of Chapters 1 through 5 you have some experience in deferring judgment. Some of these exercises asked you to produce ideas in groups without criticizing self or others.

Steps for Brainstorming

1. Appoint a facilitator. This person should be a good observer and one who can give feedback to group and its members in a helpful way.
2. Compose groups of eight to ten members. Appoint a recorder from the group if none is available to record from outside of it.

3. The facilitator should begin by making clear the two principles and four major rules of brainstorming.

4. Use *one* of the following problems as stimuli for generating ideas for all groups:

    a. how many uses can you find for a styrofoam cup?
       or
    b. how many uses can you find for a wire coat hanger?
       or
    c. how many uses can you find for a brick?

5. Brainstorm for ten minutes.

6. Following the ten minute period ask each group to count the ideas they generated. As facilitator it is important to encourage a group that had few ideas.

7. Ask group members—"what did you observe during the brainstorming process?" Encourage members to make connections between their observations and any results received from brainstorming. The facilitator also shares his observations of the process.

8. The process is then repeated with the following differences. Appoint a new recorder, lengthen the brainstorming session to twelve minutes.

9. Use the following as possible problems (choose one that all groups will use).

    a. invent different names for the term "the helping services"
    b. develop different roles for helping service volunteers
    c. find new areas of service for the helping services.

10. Ask each group to count the number of ideas they generated the second time. Were there any differences in the groups' performances between time one and time two? If so, what might they be attributed to? Have the groups comment upon any differences in their process during the second brainstorming session.

STRATEGY AND IDEA FINDING
IN CREATIVE PRACTICE

Strategy-finding is the third stage of the CPS process. As indicated in Chapter 1 what are produced in this stage are broad directions and plans for solving the problem. The strategies generated when evaluated then can be used to produce ideas for problem solution. More frequently, as demonstrated in Chapter 5, the problem solver generates a mix of both strategies and ideas to the problem definition. As an individual practitioner and not a member of an idea-finding group, say a brainstorming group, the distinction between strategies and ideas can be made more readily and put to use. The following hypothetical case example illustrates this point:

> The Winton family became involved with the Abington County Family agency because of a problem as reported by mother "of not getting along together." The worker learned from the parents and through observation of family interaction that the family had few rules for distinguishing between the roles of different family members. Parents and children were treated by all family members similarly. The parents made no demands upon their children. The Winton children constantly intruded upon the private lives of the parents.

> After several family interviews the counselor assessed the problem in this way: how can I help this family establish boundaries between the generations? The counselor then generated some *strategies*:

> 1. help the parents see the differences between their roles and their children's
> 2. model establishing boundaries for parents
> 3. encourage father to take more responsibility in the family
> 4. develop mother's incipient need to be more involved with father

The counselor, in consultation with her supervisor, decided that the second strategy, that of helping the family establish boundaries by modeling was of paramount importance.

The counselor then produced the following ideas for possible implementation in family treatment:

1. the counselor should always correct the Winton children when they interrupt their parents
2. the children should be corrected by the counselor when they are drawing attention to themselves unnecessarily
3. the counselor should tell the children that if they continue to invade their parents' bedroom in the evening they will be locked out of this room
4. the counselor will ask the parents to control their children's behavior during the family interview
5. the counselor will always let the Winton children know when they have no right to help decide specific family issues
6. the counselor will be aware of parental issues that shouldn't be discussed in the family interview and will inform the family that such issues are only to be discussed privately between the parents.

In this brief case the problem solver has produced several strategies, or general approaches for solving the problem, has chosen a single strategy and generated ideas, i.e., specific solutions, to it. Choosing more than one strategy for implementation, however, is quite legitimate. It may be important to the progress of the client system that a "strategy package" be implemented. What is true for strategies is also true for ideas. A number of ideas may be required to solve the problem. A problem solver may recognize that specific aspects of the problem take precedence over others at any one time and concentrates upon the application with the client of one solution over another. The opportunity provided by the client system situation and, of course, client need determines which ideas may be employed.

A STRATEGY AND IDEA GENERATION THEORY

Why are some individuals able to generate many fertile ideas while others appear to be "idea barren?" What motivates some persons to seek out new answers to problems while others appear comfortable with answers tested by time? Where does the creative attitude come from?

We have seen that creative theorists have attempted answers to these questions. Some, such as Rogers, Barron, MacKinnon and Maslow, have identified personality traits of creatives. Others, such as Guilford and Perkins, have sought to explain creativity through the way creatives think. Finally the psychiatric tradition has hypothesized the capacity to use regressive states, e.g., the preconscious, as explaining the creative's ability to produce imaginative ideas.

The theory that is posited here is a three factor explanation of idea generation. It takes into consideration the person but also emphasizes the psychosocial environments of the idea producer. The theory is a systems oriented explanation of idea production in that it attempts to integrate data about creative individuals coming from three sources (1) the creative person, (2) their immediate environment and (3) early psychosocial environments. Figure 25 shows the interactional nature of these factors.

Theory Factors

The person — some of the factors believed to be associated with the creative person have previously been mentioned. The factors that follow are considered critical for creative production. The creative person is one who possesses an *internal locus of evaluation*. As Rogers (1962) has presented the idea, the person draws satisfaction from the production of the idea or its materialization rather than from outside sources of approval. What this idea suggests is that the creative thinker evaluates products from an internalized set of values and principles that may be at odds with society-at-large.

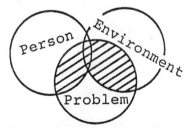

FIGURE 25. The Person-Problem-Environment theory of Idea generation.

Creative persons prefer *complexity* in problem situations (Barron, 1955). What this seems to mean is that creative thinkers may be not at all challenged or interested in relatively simple problems. *Insight*, the ability to get the point of, or to understand a situation with relatively little information, appears to be a quality of creative thinkers (Perkins, 1981). Creative persons may use insight in this way: an idea is formed by *noticing* an attribute of the solution. The total solution is suggested by the part.

Along with these qualities creative persons must be *open to experience* (Rogers, 1962). The capacity to interact non-defensively, overtly or covertly, with one's environment, and one's internally produced experience is another attribute of such persons. This openness to experience allows them to generate ideas by taking parts of their experience and by projecting upon it, to develop understandings. A defensive posture toward experience would mitigate against using a segment of experiential awareness for potential insights.

The problem — persons interact with problems that are presented by their work and interpersonal environments. Such problems can vary in the opportunity they provide the person for original idea production, as we have some problems which offer little in the way of true challenge. A helping service worker may be faced with the problem of referring a client to a service that the client clearly requires. The problem is a given and so too are the method and solution. Other problems offer greater challenge. They are not easily defined, nor when they are defined do they always present a definite method for solution.

What we may consider as a factor in promoting creative thinking is the level of problem difficulty faced by an individual. Many problems generated by certain jobs require adaptive or, as Ghiselin has called it, resourceful thinking (1964). Many on the job problems may require the reproduction of an old insight rather than the production of a new one.

Further, if job environments are to stimulate creative ideas they must promote a "tolerance for and interest in diverging views." Arieti argues that the creativogenic society must provide all kinds of divergences and that such tolerance of divergence must exist at many levels (1976, pp. 321-322). It stands to reason then that work environments must be created that illustrate such toleration, or even a fostering for divergent ways of seeing and doing so that problems can be responded to creatively. Taylor identifies a number of factors in environments that facilitate or induce creative behavior (1975, pp. 316-317). Such elements as encouragement of divergent thinking; emphasis upon problem solving and working through of conflict; general maintenance of an open environmental structure; minimization of coercion; elimination of environmental threats; allowing free communication; acceptance of fantasy and exposure to the risk-taking opinion of others are some that clearly can be connected to work environments. Such environments are more likely to stimulate interest in solving difficult problems.

Dillon has emphasized the importance of an environment that encourages students to ask questions (1982). By so doing the question asker is confronting a problem which may lead to creative idea generation.

The early environment — the environment in which we live is made up of a series of demands. As individuals we must adapt to these environmental demands or suffer at its hands. Thus, *the environment* is problematic. We learn from a very early age to cope with a variety of situations and to master them. If, as we have noted in the previous section our work environment does not provide us or allow us to work upon demanding problems, it was hypothesized, our work environment may reduce our capacity for producing creative ideas. Consider a young child's environment that offers it little in the way of life difficulties. The protective or over-protective mother may rob the young child of critical opportunities to problem solve within his environment.

MacKinnon has studied the early environment of architects who have been identified as creative (1978). There are a number of factors that suggest that the environment in which they grew provided them with the opportunity to adapt to difficult situations. He found that families of creative architects tended to move frequently, whether within a single community, from community to community or from country to country. These community and cultural dislocations were, in essence, external demands made upon the child. The form the adaptation took to these demands may have influenced the developing child's capacity for creative problem solving.

Not only did the creative architects have to cope with frequent moves to different environments they also were confronted with a family environment that differed from the norm. Parents provided these children with extraordinary respect and, as well, great confidence in their ability to behave appropriately. Such respect and confidence, it would be expected, would increase the growing children's capacity to explore the world, to make their own decisions and to express themselves freely. There often also existed a lack of closeness with one or both of the future creative's parents. An emotional distance characterized the relationship between parent and child. Such a distance, it could be suggested, allowed the child to move in his environment without experiencing the exploitation that characterizes over-dependency upon parents. Minuchin et al. in their ground-breaking work in family therapy identified two types of family structures (1967). The *enmeshed* family is one in which there are few, if any, family boundaries; because of this lack family members have great difficulty escaping from each other's excessive demands and expectations. On the opposite end of the family spectrum is the *disengaged* family, and it is a variant of this type of family structure that MacKinnon has found to be a correlate of creative development in his sample of architects. Well defined boundaries between parents and children, along with the other factors mentioned in this section, may provide a liberating effect upon the potentially creative.

Thus the childhood environment presents a set of expectations to individuals. These expectations may encourage individuals to freely explore their environment or to be inhibited in doing so. Expectations coming from the environment may promote independence or its opposite. And the environment may present cultural situations that require a form of adaptation if individuals are to develop in effective ways.

The strategy and idea generation theory presented above is a first approximation toward understanding how personal, work and familial-environmental factors work together to produce fluent and flexible ideas. Within a family environment characterized by clear expectations for responsible behavior, emotional distance and one that provides its members a multiplicity of stimuli through communal and cultural dislocations, the child responds by internalizing a locus of evaluation and an openness to experience. The child learns to prefer complexity by experiencing differing environments with differing points of view. Insight is developed through puzzling over the differences presented by a series of unique environmental experiences. Although the interaction between person and family and cultural environments produces a readiness to produce creative ideas it is only the presentation of a challenging work environment that triggers such ideas. It is the set of stimuli that the potentially creative individual must have to produce fluently and flexibly.

Summary

This chapter has introduced the strategy- and idea-finding stages of the CPS model. Strategies are broad approaches indicated for solution; ideas, on the other hand, are specific ways to solve the problem.

Brainstorming, a technique that employs important creative principles and guidelines is a valuable way to learn to internalize these principles and guidelines, and by so doing improves the user's idea-producing ability.

A strategy and idea-generation theory was introduced. This theory hypothesized the necessity of three major sets of factors for creative idea production: (1) personal elements; (2) the immediate problem-stating environment of the individual, e.g., the work environment and (3) the context that nurtured the potential idea finder.

ADDITIONAL READINGS

Sidney J. Parnes. "Toward a Better Understanding of Brainstorming," In *The Creative Process* (Ed.), Angelo M. Biondi. Buffalo, N.Y.: D.O.K. Publishers, 1972, pp. 33-45.

Sidney J. Parnes & Arnold Meadows. "Effects of 'Brainstorming' Instructions and Creative Problem Solving by Trained and Untrained Subjects." *Journal of Educational Psychology*, Vol. 50, No. 4, 1958, pp. 171-176.

Chapter 7

Strategy and Idea-Finding Techniques

There is no dearth of material on the topic of idea-finding (Figure 26). Many authors (cf. Stein, 1974, 1975; Anderson, 1980; Adams, 1974, Parnes, 1981) have written books that include procedures for stimulating creativity on an individual and group basis.

Individuals are so constructed that it would be a grave mistake to introduce them to but a few idea-finding techniques for learning purposes. Theories of creativity, as we have seen in Chapter 3, put forward distinctive factors in each theory's attempt to explain creative behavior. A theory is basically the way an individual perceives the phenomena in question. Theories differ because of differing perceptions about the phenomena. Each theory may lead to different creative practice applications. Individuals, too, differ in their perceptions of their learning needs and, as well, have different configurations of personality, attitudinal and cognitive strengths and weaknesses. Such differences indicate that it is important to present for learning a diverse group of idea-finding procedures. I have found through my teaching of CPS that individuals will strongly prefer one or several idea-stimulation methods over many others. I

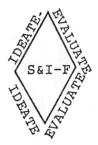

FIGURE 26. Strategy and idea-finding stage of CPS.

believe that these preferences are related to the unique personality and intellectual functioning of the individual.

Chosen for introduction and practice in this chapter are idea-finding techniques that I believe are the most productive for use in the helping services. These techniques require varied aptitudes but have the one commonality that they all demand that the user practice *deferred judgment*. Without suspending judgment the user will have the critical attitude in ascendance over the creative. The task of the idea finder is to develop quantities of new ideas; it is not to be certain or right when finding the first one. de Bono has said that the need to be right is the largest obstacle there is to defining new ideas (1977, p. 96).

BRAINSTORMING REVISITED

Brainstorming is a good technique for producing ideas in a group. It is particularly good when group members can carry out its two rules and four guidelines effectively.

Brainstorming can be complemented as a method by adding a checklist to it. We can magnify, minify and rearrange when finding ideas through the brainstorming method. By magnifying we think of ideas that are additions, increments, exaggerations and multiplications as they relate to the problem. For example look at Figure 27. We see that over time the tennis racquet has been developed by magnifying it. Once small, we now see that it has been enlarged by increasing its total size. The invention of running shoes is another magnification, one that came about by thinking of adding to shoes already in use. Increased use of spongy, shock-reducing material has been the major addition to shoes already in existence to make a running shoe. An example of a magnification in the helping service field is the use of larger units, such as the family, as the focus of treatment. The systems approach as an idea used for assessment is also a magnification. This idea allows us as helpers to gain a broad perspective in viewing a social situation. The generalist concept of the helping service worker, too, is a magnification. We now perceive the role of the worker as encompassing many more functions than was previously so.

Not only can we consider ideas that are magnifications but we can also find ideas by the use of *minification*. By thinking of ideas

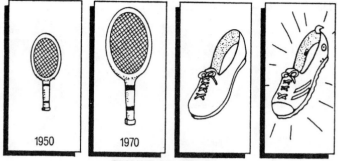

FIGURE 27. Magnify.

that divide, subtract, shorten, decrease and eliminate we find ideas that serve this function. As can be seen by Figure 28 the radio has decreased dramatically in size during the last fifty years. Short-term casework and psychotherapy are also examples of minifying ideas. Much of our society is becoming post-industrial because of a continuing minifying process. Smaller electronic components lead to a reduction in size without decrease in power of many versatile instruments. The concept of robotics is essentially a minification. As robots become more functional and "smarter" they will lead to decreases in the use of hard human labor.

By focusing upon ideas that exemplify reversals, combinations, substitutions and modifications we brainstorm by *rearranging*. Figure 29 shows that rearrangements have led to several technical innovations. The clock radio is a synthesis of the clock and radio. The van is a combination of a truck and car. The community multi-service center comes as a result of a rearranging type of idea. Rather than having services scattered throughout an urban area we have combined them for greater coordination and hopefully better service delivery. Charity organization societies were organized by recognizing the importance of coordination for cost-effectiveness.

Magnifying, minifying and rearranging are three techniques that can be incorporated into the basic brainstorming method. Before they are used, one word of caution should be made. As you learn to use these new ways to generate ideas there will be an attendant slowing down in the production of ideas as compared to the basic brainstorming technique. And this retardation is to be expected, a normal outcome of learning these new brainstorming procedures.

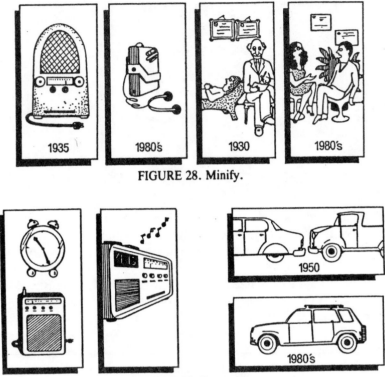

FIGURE 28. Minify.

FIGURE 29. Rearrange.

Exercise — Magnify, Minify, Rearrange

1. Form a group of eight to ten members.
2. Someone should be designated as the group leader to observe the process and to write down the ideas as they come.
3. Brainstorm for ten to twelve minutes on one of the following problems, remembering to search your minds for ideas that magnify, minify and rearrange:

   a. how can helping service workers find work in a shrinking job market?
   b. how can helping service workers identify significant problems in service delivery?
   c. how can we improve the practice education of helping service workers?

4. Discuss the total process. Share member and group leader observations with the group. Encourage the use of brainstorming rules and guidelines.
5. Repeat the process by selecting another problem. Attempt to lengthen the time used to produce ideas to fifteen minutes. Observe the process and share observations.

Exercise — A Notebook

Another way to practice magnifing, minifying and rearranging is to keep a small notebook and obsessively think about different helping service functions, processes and programs and how they might be made larger, smaller or could be combined. For example, while relaxing in a hot bath consider how group workers could minify their task of leading a group of unwed mothers. For example — by having each mother prepare to lead half a group session; by bringing in experts in parenting to talk to the group; by teaching the mothers group skills so the group functions more smoothly; by videotaping sessions without the presence of the group worker and then observing and discussing the session the following week, etc. Remember, don't judge any ideas. By keeping a notebook and jotting down various ways of magnifying, minifying and rearranging you can develop greater skill for future brainstorming sessions.

ARTIFICIAL SERENDIPITY

It is possible to find ideas by using methods that artificially introduce a random factor in our finding attempts. Several methods, although similar in form but different in label, have been developed to help us do this. Parnes (1981, p. 99) notes that *forced relationship* is a fundamental idea-finding procedure that "involves taking anything in our awareness and attempting to relate it to the problem at hand." By *anything* Parnes means that we use anything we see in our environment, images in our mind of sound, sight, taste, smell and movement, and also what we think. The techniques, of course, requires deferring judgment, for without doing so we may only select certain images or thoughts that are most *easily* related to the problem.

A similar method to that of forced relationship is de Bono's *ran-

dom stimulation. In discussing this technique de Bono declares "we use any information whatsoever." No matter how unrelated the information is it is not rejected as useless. The more seemingly irrelevant the found information is the more useful it may be to the idea-seeker (1977, p. 169).

Remember that in Chapter 4 I had identified *noticing* as an important skill for creative problem solving. Noticing is the paradoxical ability to display relaxed attention, to allow one's attention to wander from place to place in one's environment or in one's thoughts or imagination. Noticing is a way of introducing randomness into our thinking.

Therefore in order to practice *forced relationship* or *random stimulation* we must first defer judgment and secondly enter into a condition of relaxed attention, where we do not focus our attention but allow it to wander so random objects, thoughts and images may be perceived and correlated to the problem.

Introducing Randomness

de Bono has made a distinction between informal and formal randomness in the attempt to generate new ideas (1977). Informal randomness is called *exposure*. This is the act of simply putting oneself in a position where random inputs are available. We expose ourselves to them by listening receptively to other's ideas, by moving about in a large hardware store, or by allowing ourselves to be open to ideas coming from fields different from our own. We may be able to use an idea from physics, biology or computer science for solving a helping service problem.

Formal generation of random inputs is frequently required because nearly every perception we make is, in some way or another, selective. To reduce this selective factor we introduce formal methods for producing randomness in our idea-getting process. Let's scrutinize some of these mechanisms and show by example how they are used.

Method 1 —use a dictionary and randomly specify the page number, column and word number on the page you are to associate to the problem.

Problem: how can we help obese persons lose weight? A dictionary is used and the word randomly selected is *rhythmic*.

Associations:

1. Have a dance for obese persons—promotes group cohesion and self-help relationships and is also good exercise.
2. Find time of month that obese persons most easily lose weight; start them on a diet at this time.
3. Can we develop an *instrument* that obese persons can use to measure minute losses in weight (grams) to give them daily incentives for continuing on their diets?
4. Research biorhythms—is there a time of year when obese persons are at their peak physically and mentally? Is this the ideal time to begin an obese person on fitness and dietary program?
5. Encourage obese persons to identify their most enjoyable rhythmic exercise, e.g., dancing, walking, biking, swimming, etc. Encourage them to participate in it according to their level of fitness.

Method 2—walk through a library and without conscious selection pick up any book or periodical that comes to hand. Turn to a page in the book and read this chapter or, if a journal, read the article.

Problem: how can we encourage greater use of a neighborhood community center?

Associations:

1. An idea-finder randomly chose a book on photography and as she looked through it she got the idea of demonstrating the center's services by means of a slide show or photographic exhibit.
2. Another idea-finder randomly selected *Faust* by Goethe and turned to Part 1, scene 14, in which Mephistopheles tries to tempt Faust with thoughts of his beloved Margaret. The idea-finder related the scene to the word "seduction" and thought of *seducing* neighborhood residents to use the center with such events as beauty contests, dog shows and carnivals. Further, the idea-finder thought of playing *devil's advocate* by putting

out publicity flyers that challenged residents to reject the services.

3. Picking at random a novel by Karl Shapiro called *Edsel*, a third idea-finder turned to page 77 in the novel and read about the narrator's Marxist youth and how he remembered that "the first and most important trick of the Revolution . . . was to control the mimeograph machine, then the printing press, then the air waves, etc." This material easily led to the idea of a media blitz with particular focus placed upon short spot announcements on the radio. Another idea that was stimulated was to introduce a regular newsletter that would be sponsored by local merchants. Such a newsletter could give the center credibility with the residents.

Method 3 — in this method images are stimulated by playing ambiguous sounds from a pre-recorded cassette. The imager is asked to force a relationship between the received image and the problem.

Problem: the helper is intervening into the dysfunctional aspects of a marriage. Neither of the partners have surrendered their resistance to the other. Although the helper has tried various approaches to help them give up their resistance, for example, by helping them look at their communication patterns, by viewing their differences in family of origin and by assigning homework tasks, the worker has perceived scant progress in the couple's movement. The worker defines the problem this way — how can I help the male partner, who perceives having given up the most for the marriage, to reveal more about his fears, wishes and feelings to his wife?

Associations:

1. A sound is played and the worker images a fast moving train. She associates: "I open the door of the train and get the noise of the tracks. The noise is the couple's anger. S (the male partner) is not talking about his noise. The train ride is rough; the marriage is going poorly. *I must not move.* This means I must talk less, intervene less (this is a potential solution to the problem). I should keep quiet to open the door to his noise.

And the tracks are diverging. I've got to move in another direction. *I've got to go with S's resistance* (this too may be a potential solution). When he comes in and tells me how bad things are going I've got to accept that and go in his direction. That way he won't feel pressured to deny his fears and feelings."

In the last example, a worker in the apprentice stage of marital and family work uses the forced relationship technique to become aware of her blocks in working with the marital pain. The use of the ambiguous sound as a random factor triggers visual images that help her develop possible ideas for intervention with the couple.

Why does forced relationship or random stimulation or noticing work? It does so, de Bono says, because the mind works as a *self-maximizing memory system*. Two mental inputs, initially irrelevant, become linked or cohere when they are deliberately held in attention. The mind associates the two stimuli and a new relationship is formed. These idea-finding techniques, then, come as close as we can get to the serendipitous factor involved in many unique innovations, e.g., Fleming's discovery of penicillin; Goodyear's finding of the process of vulcanization and Max Ernst's discovery of frottage.

Before moving on to the next idea-finding technique, try your hand at forced relationship. Do the exercises to help improve your idea-getting ability for problem solving.

Exercise — Making the Irrelevant Relevant

Random Words

Below are listed a number of social problems that could use some creative ideas for solution. Using a dictionary ask someone to specify a page number, a column on that page and a word, for example, word 17 in that column. Using only that word that is specified force relationships between the random word and the problem. Try to find as many ideas as you can. Be confident in using this method. Remember to suspend judgment. Use the word by searching for its various meanings and by looking for directions it may take you in your thinking and by identifying what it sounds similar to.

Problems:

1. How can we raise money privately for our agency?
2. How can I find time to read one new helping service book each week?
3. How can we prevent child abuse?
4. How can we identify young families-at-risk (marital conflict, parent-child conflict, economic difficulties)?
5. How can I increase senior citizen participation in pressuring for social policy changes for their population group?

Random Objects

When we look around we notice various objects in our environment. By using these objects for forcing a relationship between it and the problem we get new ideas for solution. Practicing this idea-finding technique will develop your skill. Remember, as soon as you notice an object, whatever it is, you must try to find the relevance between it and the problem. Think of all the ways that object *might* relate to your problem. Defer judgment. Try to produce as many ideas as you can before moving on to another object.

To get you started I have listed a number of objects that might be found in a helping service agency. Use a few of these before using objects presently in your environment. Pick one of the problems listed or choose one that you wish to work on. This is an exercise that can be done on an individual basis or in a group, although it is preferable to practice forced relationship individually before using it in group situations.

Random objects:
    desk
    pen
    telephone
    intake worker
    chair

Problems:

1. How can we find conscientious and effective volunteers for a juvenile probation program?

2. How can we change the image helping service workers have as "bleeding hearts" to one more positive?
3. How can we decrease labeling and stereotyping of minorities within our local community?
4. How can we increase the chances for employability of high school dropouts?
5. How can we get ERA passed in our state?

Imaging — Our Mental Movies

Imaging can be defined as the perception of forms, colors, sounds, smells, tastes, or movement in the absence of external stimuli that could have caused such perceptions (Gordon, 1972). There is wide variation in the general population in the ability to image. Sommer has noted that some persons are anoptic, i.e., cannot image visually. He has suggested visualization training to help them improve their imaging skill (1978). Khatena, in reviewing his research on imagery and creativity, has summarized thusly:

> the more people perceive themselves as high creatives, the greater the autonomy of their imagery; that more autonomous imagers tend to produce more original images; that vivid imagers tend to perceive themselves as highly creative; that vividness of imagery tends to be related to the sense of seeing, hearing, and touching; and that in the production of original verbal images, the visual auditory and two or more of the other sense modalities are combined most frequently (1978).

It is important to be able to have control over images. Those that can control them think more divergently than those that have rigidly imposed control over their imaging (Hudson, 1966). So it seems there is some evidence linking the capacity to image with creativity. And we have already noted Arieti's idea that the image is a creative act by itself in that in its production we distort it. Our mental picture of our best friend can never be a duplicate of that person because our production of the image cannot be separated from what we feel and think about that friend at the moment we call up his or her image. The image is distorted by its emotional context. Also, the fact that images are distorted by fantasy should be stated. As an image is produced it can be elaborated by many associated images that may be determined by unconscious activity. We may fabricate and interweave a host of images that may be determined by unconscious activity. We may fabricate and interweave a host of images that make the original perception highly dissimilar to what has now been produced. Thus the ability to image and to *fantasize* can be important skills in producing unique ideas.

Not only can imaging be important for the generation of creative ideas it may also be significant for listening and understanding clients in all phases of helping service. When we empathize we are producing images that help us understand the social-emotional situation of the client. Helpers who are limited in their capacity to image may be poor empathizers in that they may disregard or dismiss certain experiences that the client relates. Not having the ability to match the client's experience with vivid imaginal production may lead to *misunderstanding* between client and helper.

Stimulating Images

A first set of techniques for producing images employs various external stimuli for eliciting them. Once the image is in awareness, forced relationship can be used to generate solutions to the problem under consideration.

I employ a series of recorded sounds, some ambiguous, others not, to trigger visual and other kinds of images. Upon playing a sound I ask listeners to attempt to image to it. Using such sounds as a thunderstorm, a freight train rolling over tracks and experimental music, listeners generate images and then attempt to force the image to the problem. For example, one student who had a great interest in marital counseling decided to work on a conceptualization of marital conflict. As the aural stimulus of the train on the tracks was played, she saw in her mind's eye the escape from an obstacle that the couple did not wish to face (resistance). She saw the obstacles as a wall made up of bricks, and the bricks in the wall represented subproblems that had to be taken down one by one in order for the conflict to disappear. She visualized a key brick that, if removed at the right time, would force the entire wall to topple. She then realized the importance of identifying the underlying problematic theme in a marital problem and intervening to resolve it.

Some individuals, upon hearing the sound that is played, may associate to the sound rather than actually produce an image. Therefore, it is important to ask the person who develops an idea from the sound how the idea was produced. What image was produced? With encouragement, and with the stipulation that images should be striven for, most individuals can generate images for ideas.

Another external stimulus used to elicit images is that of pictures of abstract art. I use slides that represent the work of Picasso, de Stael, Rothko, de Kooning and various other modern masters to help viewers creative images in various sense modalities. Essentially this is a projective technique for the viewers are perceiving images that apparently are not figurally representative and from them are creating images that come from their set of conscious and unconscious emotional and attidudinal factors. Can the use of images to produce images legitimately be called imaging? I think it can because I give the viewers the explanation that what they first see in the slide of the abstraction is not an image in the true sense; rather to make it into an image they must visually associate to this first *noticed* image and produce another one. Then this image is used to force a relationship to the problem at hand.

The artistic abstractions can be employed in varied ways to help individuals produce images. Beyond showing one picture at a time, I have used the method of quickly showing a large series of slides and then asking individuals to image to the total group what they have seen. Another way to help individuals generate images is to show abstractions in a series of two. The two abstractions are related by the viewer and then an image is produced.

Perceiving and Imaging—An Exercise

Here are two pictures of abstract art (Figure 30). This exercise will make use of them to produce images.

Begin the exercise by forming a group of at least six individuals. As a group choose a problem to which everyone can be invested. As

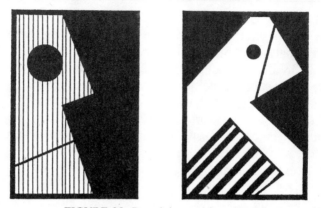

FIGURE 30. Perceiving and imaging.

a group look at the two pictures. Attempt to link them in your mind by noticing something in one of them and associating it to something else that is noticed in the other. Then image to this association. What is it that you see? Take this image and force it to the group's problem. Try, individually, to generate as many images as you can. Work on the problem as a group for ten minutes. Remember to use only *images* for forcing relationships. Defer judgment. Allow the images to surface.

Music: A Method for Releasing Images—An Exercise

Most of us enjoy a certain type of music. Whether it be folk, classical, rock, or experimental, these musical sounds can be helpful in eliciting images. These images can then be used to produce ideas for problem solving.

In this exercise we can operate individually. Find a period of time in which you will be free from interruptions. Put on a piece of your favorite music. *Relax and listen* to the music and as you do produce images to it. Spend approximately ten to fifteen minutes listening and imaging. Suspend judgment to the images you produce. Remember that creative individuals allow themselves the liberty of having external and internal experiences. Practice this exercise weekly to improve imaging ability.

Choose a problem to solve when imaging feels comfortable. Us-

ing music you find helpful for imaging begin to use the images to
force relationships between the images and the problem. Try this
for at least five minutes.

Group Imaging to Music — An Exercise

Form a group of six to ten persons. As a group choose a piece of
music that all members believe will facilitate their imaging. Then
choose a problem that needs solving, a practice problem. Produce
images to the music. Use the images to force a relationship between
them and the problem. Spend at least 10 to 15 minutes finding ideas
to solve the problem.

SYNECTICS — THE MIGHT OF THE METAPHOR (AN ADVANCED IDEA-GETTING TECHNIQUE)

Gordon, one of the discoverers of the Synectics technique, defines it as the "joining together of different and apparently irrelevant elements" (1961). These apparently irrelevant elements are
generated by a group process that supports each individual member
through a positive and non-evaluative group atmosphere. In this
atmosphere unusual and diverse elements are explored for their
value in solving a problem. Gordon gives the example of a Synectics group that was responsible for inventing a significant new product in the paint field. Rather than limiting itself to paint chemistry in
order to solve the problem, the group, made up of zoologist, physi-
cist, biologist, an artist and an engineer, considered organic cover-
ings made from seed forms of primitive plants such as algae, li-
chens, and mosses (1961, pp. 95-100).

Synectics is a problem-stating, problem-solving process. *By
making the strange familiar* (see Figure 31), i.e., understanding the
problem through exploration and analysis, the individuals composing the Synectics group convert the unfamiliar situation into a familiar one. Then the group *makes the familiar strange*. (See Figure
32.) The problem is turned upside down, sideways and in many
ways distorted to find new ways of perceiving it. The Synectics
group must be composed of persons who can understand, with help,
other disciplines' concepts and skills and comprehend the problem

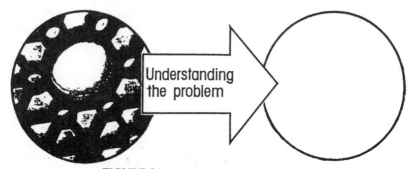

FIGURE 31. Making the strange familiar.

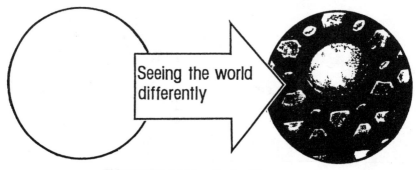

FIGURE 32. Making the familiar strange.

that requires solving. The individual requires analytic skills. Just as important, though, the individual must be able to let go of analysis and to range freely over material and to convert it into fresh ways of problem solving. To fantasize, wish for the seemingly impossible, and to imagine the non-existent are the skills required in the problem-solving phase of Synectics.

The tools that Synectics uses for making the familiar strange are *analogies*. According to Prince (1970) there are three kinds of analogies that have been found useful in helping members in a Synectics process think divergently. They are:

1. *Personal Analogy* — in this type of analogy their person identifies with the problem elements so that they can become strange. What is it like to be a poor relationship. How does it feel to be

anger? What is akin to a group that is non-cohesive? To be able to put oneself into these problems an individual must be free, expressive and spontaneous. "I am unglued and flying all around the room. I can't stay together. I'm losing my head, there's no sun to go around. I'm out of orbit. Where will I land. I'm afraid." This is a Syntectic member identifying with a non-cohesive group. The member has clearly made the familiar strange by viewing the group as a body and as a planet in the solar system. These are the ways the group as described feels to this member. Gordon gives the example of Einstein who was able to muscularly feel or empathize with mathematical ideas (1961).

2. *Direct Analogy or Example* — this tool describes the actual comparison of parallel technology, knowledge and facts. Very simply man sees a bird and attempts to build flying machines that emulate it. Or the brain is compared to a communication system that transmits signals to various parts of the body. Papanek gives the example of the bat who can find his way in darkness by using an echo location method; emitting a high-pitched sound which bounces off objects in their path, they pick up this sound with their ears and are able to avoid the obstacle-ridden path. Radar and sonar use much the same principles, radar employing ultra-high frequency waves and sonar using audible sound waves (1971). Compare the person who is depressed to a spring that has been pressed down tightly. How can we get the spring to expand to its normal size? Should we heat it? Maybe heating it is providing much human warmth. Or should it be stretched by grabbing on to its end hooks. Maybe a two-pronged approach will work. Can two persons work with the depressed? Would it be better to use individual and group therapeutic means in conjunction with each other?

3. *Book Title* — a third tool for making the familiar strange is called the book title. It is "a two-word phrase that captures both an essence of and a paradox involved in a particular thing or set of feelings" (Prince, 1970). An example of a book title is as follows:

a worker talks about a difficult client with her supervisory group. She describes the client as a very angry person who is unwilling to disclose any of this anger. "The client just sits on the lid." The group is asked to develop book titles to describe the client:

Worker 1. "I get bottled nitroglycerin"
Worker 2. "What about 'polite evil'"?
Worker 3. "Or what about 'latent violence'"?
Worker 4. "And retarded ejaculator"?

To get these book titles that attempt to combine the essence of the problem with a paradox, these workers have combined an adjective that modifies a noun. The purpose of the book title is to generalize about a particular and then to use this generality to suggest another direct analogy. For example: the leader of the supervisory group discussed above selected *latent violence* as a book title and asked the group for direct analogies from nature as comparisons. The group came up with volcanoes, the San Andreas faultline, atomic energy, and glaciers. By asking for book titles we help move the group members away from a strict adherence to the details of the problem as analyzed and toward a new direction in thinking.

Preparing for a Synectics Session

Before individual can fruitfully participate in a Synectics session they require a number of important skills.

Because Synectics is a group process that depends upon a supportive and non-critical group atmosphere it is a prerequisite that all members have experience in brainstorming, thoroughly understand and have internalized the deferred judgment guideline. The participant must also be aware of any tendencies that might prove destructive to the group process. Monopolizing, strong competitive tendencies, inability to acknowledge other member's ideas and an incapacity to empathize are all problems that would be destructive in a Synectics group.

A Synectics group, as described by Gordon or Prince, is made up of individuals from different disciplines with the purpose of each member enriching the group by contributing different kinds of knowledge and ideas. This is an ideal Synectics group and this ideal frequently cannot be met in the helping services. But a Synectics group can be composed of students or workers who have varied interests and backgrounds. Prince lists a number of worlds in an appendix of his book *The Practice of Creativity*. Such a list which, as example, is composed of such worlds as Biology, Sports, Dancing, Philosophy, Animals, Criminology, Physics, Architecture and Finance, can be used to help the group leader select members with differing backgrounds and knowledge (1970).

Finally the group members of a Synectics group must have the skills to make the strange familiar and the familiar strange. They must have a strong combination of analytic and imaginative abilities. I usually assume that it is the latter that must be learned before a member is ready for a Synectics excursion. Members must have the abilities to produce *personal* and *direct* analogies and to generate *book titles*.

Personal Analogies — An Exercise

Personal analogies require empathic identification with things or processes. Making them involves the ability to be spontaneous and expressive. We must be able to feel and to transfer such feelings into verbal expression.

Below are a number of *thing-situations*, animate and inanimate, that are a challenge to the empathizer. Use them in this way:

1. form a group of at least six persons;
2. one member should start by taking one of the *thing-situations* and attempting to identify with it;
3. other members should join in as they are able to identify with the situation. The joining in should be spontaneous; it shouldn't stand on any order within the group;
4. attempt a number of these *thing-situations* until group members feel comfortable in playing these roles.

Empathize with:

a light bulb that doesn't have filament
a breed of dog that won't bite anyone
an obese person who is dieting on 1000 calories per day
a liquid, digital watch
an apple that has no seeds
a bald snow tire

a dried-up ball point pen
a non-whistling tea kettle

Direct Analogies and Round Robin — An Exercise

Direct analogies are those things and processes that can be taken from the physical, biological and psychosocial worlds and have some similarity with the situation or problem that is confronting us.

Use a group composed of at least six members for practicing the discovery of direct analogies. Each member should take a turn at attempting to find a comparable thing or process from one of the worlds represented. If a member is unable to find an analogy, the member to the left of this group person should attempt to find a direct analogy.

Continue to go around the group until a member is able to produce a direct analogy to the problem. Present the next analogy problem to the member to the left of the group person who began the first problem. The exercise is completed when all group members have attempted a problem. Below are a number of problems that can be used to produce direct analogies.

1. Something from biological world that is similar to a pocket. For example, kangaroo pouch, mouth, cocoon.
2. Something from mechanical world that is analogous to a hat.
3. Something from physical world that is similar to constellation of the planets.
4. Something from psychological world that is analogous to death.
5. Something from biological world that is similar to a trampoline.
6. Something from biological world that is analogous to shaving cream.
7. Something from physical world that is analogous to a hammer.
8. Something from psychological world that is similar to water.
9. Something from mechanical world that is similar to a rug.
10. Something from mechanical world that is analogous to an eye.

Book Titles — An Exercise

Book titles are symbolic analogies that express a conflict between two ideas. They are formed by placing an adjective before a noun to create a tension between two ideas. For example, obesity can be seen as *generous poverty* in that the obese person certainly looks well-nourished but frequently is eating empty calories. Generous poverty illustrates an antagonism between the two ideas that may lead to further thought about the idea of obesity.

In this exercise it is important to go slowly and to allow each member in the round robin group enough time to construct book titles. Because this is a new skill the book titles that are produced initially may not be strong or provocative but with practice and with the guideline of suspended judgment firmly in mind there will be improvement.

Use the same round robin method to practice generating book titles as was employed in the direct analogies exercise. Allow each group member in turn to produce a book title from the word stimulus given. If this member cannot produce one, allow anyone in the group to attempt it. Then allow other members to join in if they are able to produce other book titles. Move to the group member to the left of the starting member for the next attempt at generating book titles.

Below is a group of words, each of which is followed by a book title. This list can be used by the round robin group as it aids its members by giving them examples in producing book titles. Following this grouping of words and book titles is a list of words that can be employed for the generation of book titles.

Anger — love's foe
Obesity — nutritional failure
Depression — unwilling passivity
Juvenile delinquency — destructive play
Suicide — successful failure
Burn Out — excessive retirement

1. rug
2. glove
3. liquid

4. tension
5. house
6. oil
7. light
8. receptivity
9. target
10. school

The Synectics Excursion

A Synectics excursion is a structured group procedure for employing the operational mechanisms that make the strange familiar and   the   familiar strange. The Synectics procedure, Prince believes, represent the problem-solving process we use daily (1970). The group moves from a lack of problem understanding to greater comprehension; a problem is defined; the group then looks for fresh ideal by using analogies; it generates ideas and determines whether these fresh viewpoints are worthwhile for attempts at problem solving.

Figure 33 is a flow chart that represents the basic structure of a Synectics excursion. Although the procedure is flexible and the use of the metaphorical mechanisms do not have to follow the exact order shown in the flowchart it is suggested that the order be followed until the leader of the Synectics session gains experience in guiding the group.

Steps in the Synectics Excursion

1. *Problem as Given* — A problem or opportunity is either handed to the group from the outside or is one that the group decides to take.
2. *Analysis and Explanation by Expert* — The expert is the person in the group who has worked on the problem and has the greatest knowledge and understanding of it. By explaining it the expert tries to make the problem clear to the other group members.
3. *Immediate Suggestions* — Group members attempt to develop possible solutions to the problem as soon as the explanation

is completed. The expert attempts to pinpoint each suggestion's values or flaws.

4. *Generation of Goals as Understood* — Each group member defines the problem as it is perceived. Goals that are desirable are wished for and imagined without constraint.

5. *Choice of Goal as Understood* — The leader chooses the goal from those formulated by the group.

6. *Leader's Question for Example* — The leader takes a keyword from the goal statement and asks group members for direct analogies to it from a particular world or field. "Can I have an example of case recording from the biological world?"

7. *Choice of Example* — From the examples generated and elaborated upon by the group, the leader chooses one that is interesting, strange and irrelevant and one for which knowledge exists in the group.

8. *Leader's Question for Personal Analogy* — The leader asks the group members to empathically identify with the example chosen.

9. *Leader's Question for Book Title* — The leader asks for two-word book titles that capture the essence of the direct analogy and is also paradoxical.

10. *Choice of Book Title* — A book title is chosen from those that are generated by the group.

11. *Leader's Question for Example* — The leader asks the group to produce direct analogies to the chosen book title. (The leader had chosen "stupid intelligence" as a book title for computer as an example.)

12. *Choice of Example* — The leader chooses an example from those produced by the group. An example from the world of biology is chosen — "instinct."

13. *Examination of Example* — Descriptive and speculative statements are encouraged to the choice of example. What is an instinct? How does it work? Who has them? Such questions may elicit a rich vein of material about the example.

14. *Force Fit* — The leader helps the members make a relationship between the material elicited by *any part of the excursion* and the goal as chosen.

15. *Viewpoint* — Relationships that are made between material

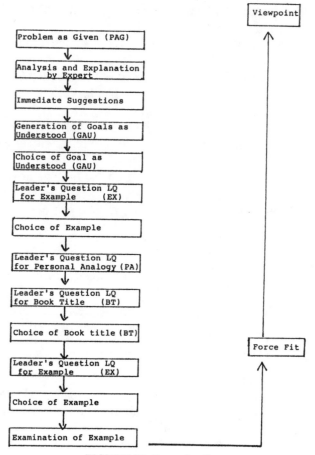

FIGURE 33. Synectics flow chart.

elicited by the excursion and the chosen goal lead to a possible solution. This solution is a viewpoint and is by no means a final solution which requires great efforts in planning and implementation.

A Synectics Excursion — An Example

A group of undergraduate helping service students illustrate the use of the Synectics process as they work on a group member's concern.

Problem as given:

Leader: So Janet wants to work on a problem she's having with a client. The client doesn't see her as competent.

Analysis and Explanation by Expert:

Janet: I've been seeing this lady now for three weeks. She's on welfare and she's been on it for a long time. Years. She's got four kids. I'm her worker now and she just won't give me the time of day. I've been straight with her, honest and all. I know I don't know what she's going thought and I admit it. It doesn't matter. She's just quietly mad. I haven't been able to reach her at all.

Immediate Suggestions:

Carla: I wonder if you couldn't show her a lot of extra warmth. Wouldn't that help?
Janet: Warmth has turned her off.
Jerry: She's angry because she has to start over with you; you're new. Couldn't you just accept the anger and realize it will go away in a while?
Janet: I think if I don't do something soon the anger will just stay with her. I've got to help her change her feelings.

Generation of Goals as Understood:

Sandy: How can we make the anger go away?
Pam: How can we take the anger away?
Janet: How can I make Mrs. X more positive about me as a worker?
Jerry: How can we change Mrs. X's anger to a positive feeling?
Carla: How can we remove the source of Mrs. X's bad feelings?
Teri: How can we make Mrs. X's life situation hopeful?

Choice of Goal as Understood:

Leader: O.K., let's try this one — How can we take Mrs. X's anger away? Let's put the problem out of our mind now.

Leader's Question for Example:

Leader: Let's see, what about an example of anger from the physical world?
Carla: Well, what about a hot springs shooting up from the earth?
Leader: O.K., that's good, any others?
Jerry: A hot, hot day. That's anger to me.
Leader: Say more Jerry.
Jerry: Well, hot weather means the sun is beating down. It's angry at us. When it's not out, it's more of a rejection.
Leader: O.K., fine. Let's hear more.
Teri: I'm thinking of a stormy sea. It's turbulent, seething, hostile.
Leader: You mean the sea doesn't want anybody near it, it's telling us to stay away.
Teri: Yeah, that's it.
Leader: O.K., let's go with the stormy sea.

Leader's Question for Personal Analogy:

Leader: As a stormy sea what do you feel? What is it like to be a stormy sea?
Jerry: Inside I feel all twisted and destructive. I'd like to get those ships and blow them apart.
Sandy: Oh, I'd like to rise higher and higher, never ending and batter myself against the shore and rocks until they give way.
Leader: Good, just beat yourself against something solid. That's anger.
Carla: I feel that I want to kill. All of my energy is going into it. I won't hold anything back. Every drop of me is being used to kill anything that comes near me.

Leader: Hey, those are really great. Let's move on from here.

Leader's Question for Book Title:

Leader: Now give me some book titles that get the essence of anger and yet are paradoxical.

Janet: Well, anger to me is the color red but what it does is turn other people off. It makes them cold or blue. What about hot turnoff?

Leader: O.K., so anger is a way to turn people off even though it is hot. What others can we come up with?

Pam: I think of anger as so exhausting. It's not worth it sometimes. But it's also necessary sometimes. We need to express it appropriately even if it may cause conflict. Maybe it's a tiring necessity.

Teri: What about emotional requirement?

Jerry: It could be a dangerous necessity.

Leader: I like that. It has tension to it. You get the conflict between the problem it could cause and its requirement for effective living.

Choice of Book Title:

Leader: Let's go with dangerous necessity.

Leader's Question for Example:

Leader: O.K., group, let's see what examples of dangerous necessity we can get from the world of biology.

Teri: I just read where bats are very important to our ecology. They pollinate fruit plants and eat insects, yet I see them as a dangerous animal.

Leader: That's a good start. What else comes to mind?

Pam: Humans, don't you think?

Leader: How do you mean, Pam?

Pam: Well, humans need each other. We've got to get along but we know we're dangerous to each other. Look at wars, murder, all the violence.

Leader: So humans are a dangerous necessity.

Carla: Bacteria. Some are fine. They live in us. But others give us sickness.

Janet: And what about the cell. We need cells to live, but sometimes they don't stop multiplying and we have cancer.

Leader: Fine, some good examples.

Choice of Example:

Leader: I'd like to examine the example of bacteria.

Examination of Example:

Leader: What do we know about bacteria? Let's look at it and see what it's like.

Teri: Bacteria are larger than a virus.

Carla: They're easy to grow too. You can set out a cheese and I think the mould that grows on it is bacteria.

Janet: Bacterial infections are easy to treat. There are a lot of anti-bacterial drugs around. I think sulfa was one of the first.

Pam: I had a strep throat once and that's caused by bacteria. They must be passed through the air and by eating food.

Leader: Anything else anyone knows about bacteria? O.K., shall we move on?

Force Fit:

Leader: Let's see, O.K., what about using that idea of bacterial infections cured by a drug. How can we fit that to our original problem—How can we take Mrs. X's anger away?

Pam: We can give her a drug. But what kind of drug takes anger away?

Carla: What's an anger-reducing emotion? Maybe Mrs. X has to really express her anger rather than holding it in.

Jerry: Yeah, she's angry but maybe she doesn't know she's angry.

Leader: Is there a viewpoint coming here?

Jerry: Sure, how about if Janet helped her to get her angry feelings out?

Leader: How?

Janet: I could bring up to her that I know she must feel

angry about losing her worker, and I could say that would make me angry.

Leader: Ah—O.K., so we've got a viewpoint. What about some others? How can we get something if we look at bacteria as easy to grow.

Janet: Well, maybe anger spreads just as easily as bacteria.

Teri: Sure, the more time spent being angry the harder it is to get rid of it.

Carla: So we just go in circles, we have to stop the anger from spreading. We know that.

Teri: But bacteria needs a particular, a receptive environment to grow.

Leader: Oh, that's good. That's more data. Let's use it.

Teri: Well, can't we change Mrs. X's immediate environment. If we do maybe some of the anger will go away.

Janet: And there's lots to change. I've talked to her about some time to herself but she won't bite on this.

Teri: But what does she want changed?

Janet: I don't know.

Jerry: So maybe you have to go after this. Find out what she wants changed and the bacteria will stop spreading.

Janet: Well, that's good. I haven't been trying to get what she wants but what I want for her, thanks, I needed that.

The Synectics excursion elicited two viewpoints that this young helping service student found helpful in her work with a welfare mother whose anger stemmed from her possible feelings of rejection and from her life situation. The student worker recognizes that the two viewpoints formulated from the excursion offer her two possible interventions that can help her reduce Mrs. X's anger and hopefully establish a good working relationship.

The Synectics method is helpful in developing viewpoints (strategies) for developing helping service inventions as well as for its use in aiding direct practitioners.

Summary

This chapter has presented a number of different strategy- and idea-finding techniques. These techniques have varied in the kind of abilities necessary for their use. A variation of brainstorming emphasizes, in the main, the cognitive ability of recall. The various methods of random stimulation rely upon such skills as associating, noticing and imaging. Synectics is a technique that requires a host of mental skills for its use. Users of this method must have a fund of knowledge at their beck and call. They must be able to use this knowledge to generate analogies. And they must be able to spontaneously express feelings as they identify with objects and processes. Finally, the Synectics user must have the capacity to *notice* relationships between the problem and the material produced through the employment of all of these skills.

The techniques that have been presented can be used to elicit strategies and ideas. As recalled strategies are broad plans and methods for achieving an end, i.e., solving a problem. Ideas are the sub-goals or the elements of a plan. The problem solver or problem-solving team must recognize whether they have produced broad or specific solutions so that the most appropriate next step in the CPS process can be taken.

The next chapter will present a method for selecting and discriminating among the strategies or ideas produced.

ADDITIONAL READINGS

Joe Khatena. *Imagery and Creative Imagination*. Buffalo, New York: Bearly Ltd., 1984.

Barry F. Anderson. *The Complete Thinker*. Englewood Cliffs, N.J.: Prentice-Hall, 1980, chapter 4.

Sidney J. Parnes. *The Magic of Your Mind*. Buffalo, New York: Creative Education Foundation, 1981.

Chapter 8

Making Decisions Creatively

Solution-finding is that stage in the CPS process at which the creative practitioner must decide on the solution most appropriate to the problem. The practitioner ends his search for strategies and ideas and focuses on choosing among them (Figure 34).

In daily life many people choose among alternatives through trial and error without considering a rationale for doing so. People use intuition to select their choice. Such methods, unsystematic as they are at times, may work. The creative practitioner, however, relies upon a systematic approach to decision-making, one that makes use of his imaginative and critical thinking faculties.

In an experimental evaluation of the decision-making process in problem solving, Nezu and D'Zurilla presented problems to individuals in three treatment conditions (1979). In the first condition instructions were given for carrying out specific decision-making procedures; in the second condition only a definition of decision-making was provided; and in the third condition, no instructions at all were given for making decisions. The investigators found that

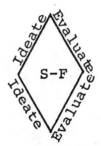

FIGURE 34. The solution-finding stage of CPS.

the results supported their hypothesis that instructions in decision-making procedures enhanced decision-making ability. A further study by the same investigators confirmed these results (1981). This evidence suggests that training in decision-making enhances this ability.

DECISION-MAKING FOR HELPING SERVICE PRACTICE

Making decisions is a critical skill in problem-solving behavior (D'Zurilla & Goldfried, 1971). A problem-solving practice demands that the problem-solving practitioner have an effective methodology for making decisions and alternatively demonstrate to clients how this methodology can be learned and used in everyday life. As shown by Nezu and D'Zurilla decision-making can be enhanced through instruction. Then it is crucial that practitioners know how to guide clients in learning this set of decision-making skills (1979; 1981).

Many practitioners in various forms of helping practice encourage their clients to reflect on the possible consequences of various alternative forms of action. Hepworth and Larsen, in an approach which they specifically label as problem-solving practice, offer this procedure as part of an effective means for improving decision-making ability (1982). The Nezu and D'Zurilla evidence, however, suggests that a systematic approach to decision-making facilitates making good decisions. For example, in evaluating consequences they ask decision-makers to consider four categories of outcome as criteria:

> short-term, long-term, personal (i.e., effects on oneself), and social (i.e., effects on others and the community). In estimating likelihood, there are two considerations. One is the likelihood of a particular course of action producing a particular effect on the individual and/or the social environment in question. The second is the likelihood that an individual confronted with the problem will be capable of implementing the particular course of action effectively, which requires an assessment by the problem-solver of possible obstacles and resources in

the social environment, as well as an evaluation of his own personal assets and liabilities. (1979, p. 270)

Considering and reflecting upon the criteria that Nezu and D'Zurilla indicate as important for decision making is a significant part of their decision-making procedure. A major difference between their approach to decision-making and the solution-finding stage in CPS is this: in solution-finding the criteria used for evaluating solutions are *not* indicated by the CPS model. Because the model emphasizes *creative* problem solving any criterion may be considered and selected for the evaluation of potential solutions. As I will indicate later there are other criteria that can fall outside of the categories suggested by Nezu and D'Zurilla above.

PREPARING FOR EVALUATION

Solution-finding begins when we have ordered or categorized the strategies and ideas generated in the idea-finding stage. Anderson has identified three factors that must be considered for this task (1980). The set of solutions to the problem must be:

1. complete;
2. minimal, and
3. non-redundant.

By *complete* Anderson means that all important solutions are included. Clearly we can never know that our package of strategies or ideas is complete. Time may constrain us from producing as many ideas as we can. The importance of the problem also plays a part in the completeness of our solutions. Is the problem one to which we are deeply committed or are we willing to accept a set of solutions quickly arrived at? Or does commitment have little to do with completeness? A serious problem faced by a client may demand a relatively quick solution without benefit of leisurely search for solutions. Completeness then is a subjective belief that we have produced a set of alternatives compatible with the seriousness of the problem *and* the amount of time at our disposal.

Solutions produced are minimal if they include no *unimportant* ones. Therefore, prior to the solution-finding stage we screen the strategies or ideas produced in these stages. We scrutinize strategies produced, and through group discussion or careful individual judgment, we exclude those that are obviously not good. The same procedure is followed for ideas. Idea-finding techniques are helpful in generating quantities of strategies and ideas. Clearly, however, such a large number must include many that have little value as potential problem solutions.

A third factor that must be considered before criteria are produced for decision-making is that of redundancy. Redundant solutions are those that are essentially not different from each other. Let's take an example of a set of solutions that does illustrate redundancy. In an attempt to evaluate my course in CPS I asked students to respond to problem situations with as many ideas that they could produce in a five-minute period. Below is the problem situation and the students' ideas for solving it.

Problem:

Dawn Williams is 35 years old and has been married eight years. Until this year she has been happily married. Lately, there has been a change in the behavior of her husband, Charles, age 34. Although most of the time his behavior is normal, he sometimes has outbursts of anger and aggression.

Solutions:

Leave temporarily
Leave permanently
Get counselling
Find support group
See doctor
Go to family service
Go to priest
Go to police
Use friends for support
Talk to boss
Go to Children's Aid
Go to A.A. for support

As can be seen, although the student has produced a good quantity of ideas for the time allotted, many of the solutions are redundant. Many of these solutions would fall under the rubric of getting counseling and advice from an external source. Because a long period of strategy- or idea-finding can produce a large quantity of solutions it is important to identify those that can be eliminated on the basis of redundancy. Care must be taken to understand the meaning of each strategy or idea after their generation. Although a solution may be worded differently from another there may be no difference between them. Consider the problem of how to improve employment opportunities for youth. One solution that might be produced to this problem is *to insure that programs are available for the improvement of job-related skills for at-risk youth.* Another solution produced to this problem is *to insure that at-risk youth get the vocational training necessary to make them enjoyable in today's job market.* As can be seen both solutions are identical, for they both call for training *necessary* for employment. Although couched in different language both solutions are equivalent. The problem solver must be aware of redundancies when sorting out solutions in preparation for decision making.

Exercise — Excluding the Losers

Convene a group that has produced a large number of strategies or ideas. Identify good ones from the poor by holding a brief discussion of each of them. Spend thirty seconds to a minute discussing each of them. This time limit will be difficult to maintain; therefore, appoint a member from the group to monitor the group's discussion on each. The size of the strategy or idea pool will determine the length of time spent on this exercise. If the pool is of a moderate size, say twenty or so ideas, the exercise should take approximately 12 to 15 minutes.

SORTING STRATEGIES AND IDEAS

You have had the experience, if you became involved in the idea-finding exercises, of generating large quantities of possible solutions to a problem. Such a group of solutions does not always fit neatly into a group of strategies nor does it into a group of ideas; rather, it is highly likely that a mixed group of both has been produced. I have said that the modified CPS model contains a strategy-

and-idea-finding stage, and, as well, two solution-finding stages. These solution-finding stages are necessary for deciding on strategies as well as the ideas generated to these strategies. Because it is so difficult to generate *only* strategies or *only* ideas while producing alternatives for solution it is critical that following such production the practitioner sort the solutions into their appropriate groups. Remember, *strategies* are broad plans and directions to reach a goal. *Ideas* are specific, and may or may not relate to a strategy. Evaluating a large number of solutions without recognizing the difference between them as either strategies or ideas can cause the practitioner much confusion. Strategies and ideas may be lumped together for decision-making rather than first deciding to develop either a strategy or set of strategies. When the strategy has been determined it is time to generate ideas with idea-finding techniques. Ideas initially produced in the first alternative generation stage are included in this group if they relate to the strategy decided upon.

The following hypothetical example illustrates the process of using two alternative generation and two decision-making stages as described above:

> A marital couple request sexual counseling at a mental health center. Based upon a definition of the problem the practitioner indicates two directions for treatment: increasing sexual intimacy and improving communication between the couple. Relating to sexual intimacy both practitioner and both partners produce numerous ideas. They decide upon a weekend vacation to help them relax. Many ideas are then produced for implementing the communication strategy. The couple decide upon implementing the following: increasing their talking time in the evening, and encouraging each other to talk about their jobs.

Figure 35 depicts the process of generating strategies and ideas, selecting strategies, generating ideas for them and then selecting ideas for implementation.

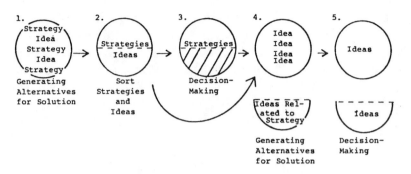

FIGURE 35. The process of generating solutions and deciding among them.

Exercise — Redundancy

Convene a group that has generated a large number of alternatives for solution. Then, as a group:
1. identify solutions that are *strategies*;
2. identify solutions that are *ideas*;
3. group solutions that are similar in content. Discuss these solutions within the group and determine whether they have distinguishing features or are equivalent as strategies or ideas.

THE DECISION-MAKING DILEMMA

The creative problem solver, when involved in the decision-making process, finds himself in a serious dilemma. The problem solver is bound, on the one hand by the Charybdis of *utility* and, on the other, by the Scylla of *probability*. Utility can be defined as the *desirability of the expected consequences of an action*. Utility connotes effect. It is the desired impact that a *solution* may have upon a problem. Naturally, as helpers, we want to choose highly utilizable solutions. But we also have to consider *probability — how likely is it that the expected consequences of using the chosen solution will be the result*. As Bloom has noted, both factors can vary independently (1975). What we want to happen may not have any chance of being implemented. Alternately, there may be a very strong chance that what we place little value upon may readily be implemented. For example, a working couple who are experiencing difficulty in agreeing upon child-rearing decide they will spend one hour discussing their actions after putting the children to bed. This solution is viewed by the couple and the worker as highly desirable. Unfortunately, the couple find they are too tired to follow through. They decide, instead, to provide each other with a recorded cassette of their daily thoughts on their respective actions as parents. Although this may be a feasible solution the impact that it can have on their problem will, mostly likely, be low. Figure 36 depicts the possible relationships between the utility and probability factors.

Bloom contends that "decisions often mean practical compromises between some combination of utility and probability" (1975). In day-to-day helping service practice this guideline makes sense. I would like to offer a caveat, however, against making this guideline into a dictum. Frequently, a highly utilitarian idea, i.e., a creative one, is forsaken because the individual or group considers it improbable, without significantly studying the factors that may mitigate its implausibility. Our judgment of solutions of great potential is frequently harsh. This, too, makes sense. The obstacles to implementing truly creative ideas are formidable. The world we live in is complex. Frequently, we professionals are faced with undeniably difficult funding problems. Administrative difficulties may abound. Yet if we are to innovate in the helping services these are exactly the kinds of challenges that we must confront. Creative

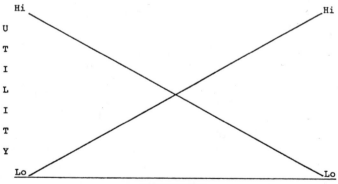

FIGURE 36. Relationships between utility and probability as decision-making factors.

ideas must not be neglected because they appear, upon first glance, to be unworkable.

CRITERIA FOR DECISION-MAKING

In this section I will explore the use of *criteria* for choosing among strategies and ideas. Criteria are those factors that are used in the *evaluation* of generated strategies and ideas. For example, consider a social agency that has this concern: its waiting list for service is growing larger each month. It determines that the problem it must solve is the reduction of the list without reducing service delivery effectiveness. A number of strategies for doing this are generated. Agency staff think of:

1. developing a screening device to determine who most clearly needs to be served first;
2. organizing a group program to support people until they receive individual help;
3. attempting to negotiate a change in the agency's catchment area so fewer individuals apply for service;
4. developing a family life education program for those that presently receive family treatment but are assessed as able to benefit from an educative approach; and
5. organizing groups comprised of families for inter-family therapy sessions.

What criteria should this agency use to determine which of these alternatives can best solve its problems? The agency administrator quickly thinks of *costs*. How much money must be allocated to make these solutions operational? Another staff person thinks that *resources* must be used as a *criterion*. Are there enough staff to carry out these alternatives? And what about *impact on the objective*? Which of these solutions will have the greatest effect on the problem? Which solution is most *feasible*? Are there some alternatives that present far too many obstacles to their implementation?

As can be seen there are any number of criteria that can be framed for evaluating these strategies. How are these criteria established? Some come to mind *logically* as the problem, the alternatives for solution and the context of the problem are reflected upon.

The Function Complex

Victor Papanek, winner of the Nobel prize for design, uses what he calls the *function complex* for determining good design (1973). By design Papanek means "the conscious effort to impose meaningful order." For him design includes such efforts as composing a poem, executing a wall mural or writing a symphony. It can also involve, he says, pulling a tooth, baking a pie, cleaning and reorganizing a file and educating a child. Using Papanek's definition of design we can see that helping service practice, where we are using knowledge of theory and technique, *is* design. Good design depends upon the interaction of a number of criteria that Papanek has labelled the *function complex* (Figure 37).

The following are the elements of the complex:

1. *Use*—by use is meant whether the design will work effectively. This functional criterion is closely related to the one called *effect on objective*. But Papanek goes further than asking that a design work. He asks: how can we know about the future effects of this design? What may be its unintended consequences? As example, Papanek points to the automobile, with its polluting, its ability to kill thousands of persons each year, its generation of exurban sprawl, and attendant network of highways that cost governments huge sums of money.

    Another example is the building of large mental hospitals or asylums in the latter part of the 19th century. When a person

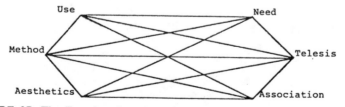

FIGURE 37. The Function Complex. Used with the permission of Victor Papanek, *Design for the Real World* © 1973, Pantheon Books, a division of Random House, Inc.

was judged insane he was placed in these institutions. His chance of leaving it in better health was slim. Why? Because it was not recognized at the time that institutionalization in itself fostered, in most cases, the illness (Goffman, 1961).

As designers of new procedures, programs and social legislation helping service professionals must be acutely aware of not only such programs workability but also what the unintended consequences of their use will be. This is no easy task. However, thoughtful reflection on the use of helping service methods may prevent serious problems from emerging in the future.

2. *Method* — method is defined as the interaction of tools, processes and materials. Poor method results from a misapplication of these elements. The helper has at her command a number of tools and processes for good design. The builder may use studs and joists for material; hammer, nails and saw for tools and various "joining" processes for tying the materials together. The helper uses her *self* as tool and such processes as problem solving as practiced within various system contexts. Completing the analogy, the client is the material in the helping service domain. Individuals who come to us for help are the material to which we apply our processes and tools. A misapplication of our self and our processes to the material (our clientele) will result in poor design. And, in part, good design depends upon the clientele we ply our tools and processes upon. Good method in the helping services is highly dependent upon a good fit between tools, processes and materials. All practitioners have experienced the frustration attending the inability to help someone with the tools and processes that make up their professional expertise. Therefore, method, as an evaluative criterion, causes the practitioner to reflect upon the correlative fit between her self, her processes and her clientele.

3. *Aesthetics* — aesthetics is that functional criterion that is used to consider the beauty, elegance and balance of a design. A work of art is primarily judged on its aesthetic quality. Does helping service practice, procedure, program and policy require judgment on an aesthetic level? Consider what is meant

by an elegant solution. It is one that has been reduced from a state of complexity to one of simplicity. A new creation frequently draws the response — "why, that's so simple, so clear." The solution appears to be within everyone's grasp once it has been realized. The creator has seen clearly through the complex of factors imbedded in and surrounding the problem to the heart of the matter. Practitioners *should* appreciate the aesthetic yardstick in evaluating their creations.

Helping service techniques should be clear, precise and understandable. Empathic understanding, used to build a trusting and helping relationship and to further client exploration of self, is such a technique. It consists of a number of clearly identified sub-skills, verbal and non-verbal. The food stamp program is an aesthetic one, in that it is a fine solution to the problem of lack of food money. Providing food for those who do not have it is a clear, simple and elegant solution.

4. *Needs* — a need satisfies the physical, economic, psychological, intellectual or spiritual aspects of a human being. When helpers require good design they must distinguish between needs and wants. Wants are those desires built and manipulated by a consumer-oriented society. Practitioners, such as adoption workers, may be impressed by the social status of aspiring adoptive parents rather than carefully scrutinizing their parental qualities. Practitioners may *want* to work in prestigious agencies where the need may not be as great as in the public services. Or they may want private practice after their educational stint because of its high status connotations (Falck, 1984). Helping service practitioners, then, are not immune to designing procedures, programs and policy that reflect the consumer-orientation of their society. Need can be a critical yardstick in the selection of well-designed strategies and ideas.

5. *Telesis* — this is the purposeful correlative fit between natural and societal goals. A design should reflect the socioeconomic times and conditions that have given rise to it. Practicing psychoanalytic treatment as if all clients in North America were hysterical refugees from late 19th century Vienna is an exam-

ple of such a lack of fit. Building public housing units, clearly visible as such, in undesirable ghetto areas, is a good example of a lack of correlative fit between the societal goal of integration and housing need. Such practice only leads to stigmatization in a purportedly democratic society. Social programs that reflect the values and practices of past socioeconomic conditions, such as those that encourage the dependency of the aged, are non-teletic in design. Design of procedure, program and policy frequently represents a compromise between societal groupings, some of whose ideas and values conflict with others. The teletic criterion can help the practitioner be alert to the danger of design that does not correlate with present social conditions.

6. *Association* — closely allied to the criterion of telesis is that of association. By association, Papanek means the effect our individual history, e.g., attitudes, values and traits, have upon our actions. An example of association operating in design is the television set. Designers still have not made up their minds whether it is a recreational device or a piece of furniture and, in many instances, it is combined into both. Many practitioners trained in the era dominated by psychoanalytic theory view clients in terms of pathology alone, without considering their strengths and positive capacities. Association also operates by determining in helping service practice whether helpers view social phenomena as a result of basic *cause and effect*, or as a systemic interaction. The complexity of social interaction, as exemplified by the many factors that may effect a family conversation, e.g., context, family size, topic of conversation, time of day, emotional configuration, etc., would strongly suggest the use of systems perspective for analysis. Yet, because of associational factors many helpers still cling to a deterministic position.

As can be seen the function complex offers the helping service practitioner *one* set of criteria for use in judging possible solutions (designs). Added to those criteria discussed in our example of the social agency with an extended waiting list, i.e., those of cost and resources, we see that there *can* be many yardsticks used for decision-making. Many more can be produced in the ideation phase of solution-finding. Those criteria most potent for decision making are determined by the problem under consideration.

Exercise — Producing Yardsticks

In a group, using any problem that the group wishes, generate strategies and ideas relating to it. Spend 10-15 minutes in the idea-finding stage. Following this stage produce as many yardsticks for evaluating these potential solutions as you can. Remember to defer judgment as you did in the idea-finding stage. Go beyond the function complex in your efforts. Try for at least 12-15 potential criteria.

Deciding on Yardsticks

We are ready to evaluate strategies and ideas when we have ordered the solutions produced in the strategy/idea-finding stage of CPS and when we have followed this with the generation of *criteria* to judge this group of solutions. Let's take an example.

A helping service student is interested in the anger of children between the ages of six to ten and who have shown some emotional disturbance. She frames her problem thus: how can I encourage children at this age level to express angry feelings appropriately? Some of the solutions she produces are:

1. developing a group discussion format for working on the problem with children;
2. working with the children individually in an approach similar to play therapy;
3. discussing emotions and how to deal with the anger emotion in the classroom;
4. using myths, fairy tales and fables as a way to elicit discussion in school or an informal setting;
5. working with the parents of the children so they may teach their children appropriate methods of dealing with anger;

6. using television as a medium to illustrate situations in which anger is appropriately and inappropriately used; and
7. using plays to illustrate situations of anger.

The student recognizes that nearly all of her solutions are different from each other. Solution 1 and 3 are similar. She also notices that the solution most clearly an idea is solution 4. She categorizes the rest of the solutions as strategies. Following this procedure the student produces these criteria:

1. resources needed
2. effect on objective
3. telesis
4. ethicality
5. method
6. time
7. effect on people
8. effect on future
9. aesthetics

When she had compiled this list of yardsticks for deciding on a solution her next step was to turn them into *clear and specific criteria* related to the problem, her solutions and the problem's context. To do so she produced *criteria-spurring questions* to each of the criteria. In so doing she employed *deferred judgment*. Below are the criteria-spurring questions she generated to each yardstick:

1. *Resources needed* — how much money will I need to effect this solution? What expertise will I need to complete the solution?
2. *Effect on objective* — what solution would bring the most lasting effect? When is it most effective to achieve the objective? What other positive changes might the solution bring about?
3. *Telesis* — what solution makes the most sense, to children, given today's social conditions?
4. *Ethicality* — what solution would best fit with parental values? What social institutions might object to those solutions?
5. *Method* — what process would best fit the material, i.e., the children? Effectively, how long should the process be?

6. *Time* — what solution requires the most time to implement? How can I implement a solution given that I have six months to do so?
7. *Effect on people* — who might have difficulty using it? Who might misunderstand the solution's intention? How might it change parental practices?
8. *Effect on future* — how might it produce unintended consequences? What improvements might the solution need in the near or distant future?
9. *Aesthetics* — what solution embodies best the quality of logical simplicity? What solution would be most appealing to the implementor? To the children?

The helping service student then transformed these questions into yardsticks that she could use to judge her solutions. The following are the concepts she made from her questions:

1. Resources needed

   a. money accessibility*
   b. accessibility to expert resources

2. Effect on objective

   a. lasting impact*
   b. appropriate implementation time
   c. unintended consequences of solution

3. Telesis

   a. solution appropriateness

4. Ethicality

   a. solution-parent value fit
   b. solution rejection potential

5. Method

   a. process appropriateness
   b. right method length

6. Time

   a. time cost
   b. allotted time for solution*

7. Effect on people

   a. user difficulty in implementing solution
   b. solution understandability
   c. impact on parental behavior

8. Effect on future

   a. unintended consequences
   b. solution modifications in future

9. Aesthetics

   a. solution elegance
   b. solution fit with user
   c. solution fit with clientele*

The student has produced twenty criteria by asking criteria-spurring questions, obviously too many to encounter in evaluating the solutions. She pares these down to four by identifying those she considers most important for the decision-making process. (This selection of the critical yardsticks would be completed through a give-and-take discussion if done in a group.) She chooses:

1. money accessibility
2. lasting impact
3. allotted time for solution, and
4. solution fit with clientele

In choosing these four yardsticks for decision making the student recognizes that in the group of twenty she has created are some that are similar to each other. Therefore her task in choosing criteria most relevant for decision making is made easier by eliminating these duplicates. The student knows that without money she would be unable to carry out the solutions she has produced. And she wants a solution that will have lasting effect upon the problem. She knows also she must work within her time limit, eliminating those that cannot be finished within the six months she has for development and implementation. Finally, the student recognizes that the solution must closely fit her target group, those children between six and ten.

USE OF IMAGINATIVE AND EVALUATIVE THINKING

The helping service student has used both imaginative and evaluative thinking in generating criteria for use in decision making. Producing broad criteria such as *resources needed, method* and *effect on objective* is followed by producing criteria-spurring questions to them. Since *any* question may be asked we employ deferred judgment in this task. Once questions have been generated to each of the broad criteria our task is to *abstract* from the question a specific concept that is to stand on a lower level of generality than did the first group. Figure 38 depicts this movement from broad to more specific criteria. What must be kept in mind is that forming these concepts is a creative act that requires practice before it becomes a skill for use in decision making. The concepts formed in this process are neither right nor wrong. They are inventions formed by creative thinking.

Exercise — Conceptualizing by Producing Criteria-Spurring Questions

Either individually or in group change the questions generated for producing criteria into more specific conceptual criteria.

The *problem* is: *how can we educate our helping agency about the problem of burnout?*

The Solutions:

1. Send a letter to each agency staff about the dangers of burnout;
2. Have a workshop on burnout;
3. Have a speaker lecture on burnout in the agency;
4. Develop a multi-media slide and tape show illustrating the problem and its remedies;
5. Produce a videotape on the problem and its possible solutions;
6. Organize an agency day where all agency staff attend and discuss the problem;
7. Read books on burnout;
8. Develop a package that includes literature, film, speakers

and experiential workshop;

9. Develop a helping service course on organizational problems that includes the topic of burnout;
10. Organize a panel of burned out helpers who have combatted the problem and who come to our agency to educate workers.

The Criteria:

costs —
1. Do we have money to develop and implement solutions?
2. What solution is cheapest?
3. How can money be recouped to meet project costs?
4. Are there ways of raising money for the projects?

resources —
1. Do we have expertise to implement solutions?
2. What is the solution most readily implemented, given our present skill?
3. What expertise can we recruit for minimal expense?

time —
1. Can we complete the project within a year? What solutions may be implementable in the near future?

effect on objective —
1. What solution will give the social worker the necessary amount of data to enable them to cope with burnout?
2. What solution would have greatest impact?

telesis —
1. What would be the most appropriate media to use in educating helpers?

need —
1. What solution meets the most immediate need of social workers?

ethicality —
1. What solution might helpers reject because it/they intrudes/intrude upon personal or professional value systems?

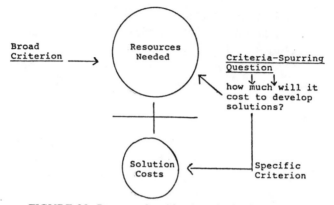

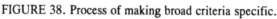

FIGURE 38. Process of making broad criteria specific.

2. Are there solutions that intrude upon the administrative mandate of the agency?

method —   1. What process fits best with educating helpers about burnout?

The Concepts:

costs —   1. _____
    _____
    2. _____
    _____
    3. _____
    _____
    4. _____
    _____

resources —   1. _____
    _____
    2. _____
    _____
    3. _____
    _____

time —   1. _____
    _____

effect on objective – 1. _____

2. _____

telesis – 1. _____

need – 1. _____

ethicality – 1. _____

2. _____

method – 1. _____

USING CRITERIA FOR CREATIVE DECISION MAKING

The Evaluation Grid

So far the solution-finding process has involved the following steps:

1. The generation of broad categories of criteria;
2. The production of criteria-spurring questions to each of the broad criteria;
3. The transformation of these questions into concepts that represent specific criteria; and
4. the selection of a number of these conceptual criteria based upon their relevance for application to the group of solutions.

How many criteria should be selected for decision making? My experience has helped me form a rule of thumb. Using more than five criteria for decision making, particularly in groups, becomes tedious and unproductive. Decision-makers tire and become confused. With fewer than three criteria for evaluation the decision-making process lacks power. The decision-makers, in all likelihood, have eliminated an important criterion from the evaluation process. Therefore, in evaluating solutions I suggest using no fewer than *three* criteria and no more than *five*.

The *evaluation grid* is a tool that should be used flexibly to make decisions between solutions. By flexible I mean that the results of the decision-making process should not be considered final or irrevocable. Let's consider the following example of the evaluation grid's use.

A helping service agency has decided to buy a microcomputer to assist in the agency's administrative tasks. The staff has decided that the following criteria are the most relevant in choosing between five microcomputers:

1. ease of use
2. durability
3. software accessibility, and
4. availability of service and maintenance.

As a group of six staff they meet and construct an evaluation grid (Figure 39).

Following the construction they agreed to rate each of the computers on all four criteria chosen. They decided that if as a group they agreed that a computer was *outstanding* on a criterion, it would receive a rating between 8-10; if *good* it would be assigned a rating of 6 or 7; if *fair* a rating of 4 or 5; and if *poor* it would receive anything in the range of 1 to 3.

IDEAS	EASE OF USE	DURABILITY	SOFTWARE ACCESSABILITY	AVAILABILITY OF SERVICE AND MAINTENANCE
Byte 1				
Super Concorde				
Flying Dynamo				
Excessively Friendly				
Great Data Bank				

FIGURE 39. An evaluation grid.

The group then discussed each computer as it related to each criterion. Ratings were finally assigned. The results of this procedure are shown in the completed evaluation grid (Figure 40).

What has the group accomplished? It has, through the evaluation procedure, determined that there are two computers, the Flying Dynamo and the Great Data Bank that do not meet the computer needs of the agency. But what about the other three computers? Is Excessively Friendly the best computer for the agency? It did rate highest among the five computers that were evaluated. Or does the fact that Excessively Friendly, Byte 1, and Super Concorde, the three most highly rated computers respectively, were but a few points apart suggest that further evaluation is required?

Consider this possible problem: might there be one evaluation criterion that the group believes should be weighted more heavily than the others? For example, does software accessibility, i.e., the capacity of the computer to accept various computer applications, require a greater value than the other three criteria? If so, it may be necessary to evaluate the computers to take into account this greater value.

THE METHOD OF PAIRED COMPARISON

How can we determine the value to be placed on criteria used in the decision-making process? The *method of paired-comparison* can help those involved in the process determine the ratio of weighting between criteria.

IDEAS	EASE OF USE	DURABILITY	SOFTWARE ACCESSIBILITY	AVAILABILITY OF SERVICE AND MAINTENANCE	TOTAL
Byte 1	5	9	4	8	26
Super Concorde	7	6	5	7	25
Flying Dynamo	4	5	5	3	17
Excessively Friendly	9	7	6	6	28
Great Data Bank	5	3	8	5	21

FIGURE 40. Completed evaluation grid.

Let's again consider the example of choosing between five computers with the aid of four criteria. To begin the paired-comparison technique all criteria are listed and then *evaluated against each other*. Remember that our criteria for use in deciding upon a computer are:

1. ease of use
2. durability
3. software accessibility, and
4. availability of service and maintenance.

We compare these criteria to each other and determine which between the two is most important., By doing so we are able to obtain a count of how many times one criterion is considered more important than any other. By doing this we are establishing *weights*, or differing values for each criterion. This process for the four criteria is shown below.

Criteria	Comparison	Decision
1. Ease of use	1. ease of use vs. 2. durability	ease of use (1)
	1. ease of use vs. 3. software accessibility	software accessibility (3)
	1. ease of use vs. 4. availability of service and maintenance	ease of use (1)
2. Durability	2. durability vs. 3. software accessibility	software accessibility (3)
	2. durability vs. 4. availability of service and maintenance	durability (2)
3. Software accessibility	3. software accessibility vs. 4. availability of service and maintenance	software accessibility (3)

The result of our comparison analysis is the following:

1. ease of use − 2
2. durability − 1

3. software accessibility — 3
4. availability of service and maintenance — 0

Based upon this analysis we assign weighting factors as follows:

— software accessibility   = 3
— ease of use   = 2
— durability   = 1
— availability of service and maintenance   = 0

How do we determine which criterion is most important when we make comparisons between them? In a group this is done through a discussion using analytic reasoning. When deciding on our own, we must rely upon careful reasoning and judgment without benefit of any corrective feedback from group members.

Following the determination of weights for each criterion, a *scale* is selected for use in deciding how each solution measures up to another. For demonstration purposes we can choose a scale that uses four simple values;

— excellent   = 4
— good   = 3
— fair   = 2
— poor   = 1

The evaluation grid is then used to evaluate the solution, employing the weights determined for each criterion factor and the scale values to be given each solution. The grid is modified to accommodate for these uses. As shown in Figure 41, the criterion score for each solution is multiplied by the weighting score. For example: Byte 1 has received a criterion score of 2 (fair) for ease of use. This score is multiplied by its weighting of 2 to arrive at a score of 4. This procedure is repeated for all four criterion factors. Then we use the same computational procedure for each potential solution.

When the results of the first evaluation are compared with the second, employing the paired-comparison method, we notice several differences. First, we note that we have new leaders. The Great Data Bank, based upon the weight given to the software accessibility criterion and the computer's high rating on this value, has pulled

IDEAS	CRITERIA					
	ease of use	durability	software accessibility	availability of service and maintenance		
	WEIGHTING FACTORS					FINAL
	2	1	3	0	TOTAL	ACTION
Byte 1	2(4)	4(4)	2(6)	4(0)	14	
Super Concorde	3(6)	3(3)	2(6)	3(0)	15	
Flying Dynamo	2(4)	2(2)	2(6)	1(0)	12	
Excessively Friendly	4(8)	3(3)	2(6)	2(0)	17	
Great Data Bank	2(4)	1(1)	4(12)	2(0)	17	

FIGURE 41.

even with Excessively Friendly. Byte 1 and Super Concorde have changed their positions in the evaluation, although numerically there is little difference between them. Flying Dynamo still is considered to be a poor risk by our decision-making group. The differences that can be seen between the two separate evaluations are related to two major factors: (1) that software accessibility was considered to be the criterion of utmost importance to the group, and (2) that availability of service and maintenance was thought to be of relatively little importance.

What do our helping service decision-makers do now. Certainly they can't buy two computers, not in this era of financial restraint. They must decide between the two computers based upon the group's collective judgment. Although both computers received equal numerical value it may be most important to the agency that the Great Data Bank has greater potential for applicability than does Excessively Friendly.

We should be aware that solutions that have been evaluated equally may be made into a *solution-package*. Several solutions may be used to creatively solve a problem. Because social problems are so resistant to intervention it may be relevant to work on them from several different directions. Decision-makers in the solution-finding stage of CPS should be highly aware of the possibility of using more than one solution to solve a problem.

DECISION MAKING BY TECHNIQUE: A CAVEAT

We have discussed solution-finding by evaluating solutions through the process of developing criteria and assigning ratings to them. In the case of the paired-comparison method we have illustrated how these criteria can be weighted, showing the esteem in which they are held by decision makers. These are valuable techniques for evaluation, for frequently we may decide without consciously being aware of the reasons we hold for making important decisions. *But we must not become overly enamored of the seemingly precise numerical data that we generate in these processes.* We must be aware that the numbers that we assign to each criterion are made only as objectively as human beings can. There is, of course, bias, prejudice and irrationality present in any rational procedure. A rational decision-making process can only hope to *control* these factors. It should be recognized that the numerical precision that can be gained by decision-making techniques is no substitute for the good judgment that stands behind them.

Summary

The solution-finding stage of CPS is a decision-making stage. It makes use of the generation of broad criteria and the specification and selection of these criteria for use in deciding among alternative solutions. Papanek's function complex, as well as the logic of the problem solver, offers suggestions for the broad criteria initially to be considered for evaluating solutions. By employing deferred judgment, the problem solver generates criteria-spurring questions that help in the transformation of broad to more specific criteria. Selection of these criteria most relevant for judging the solutions is followed by the use of rating and weighting techniques. Such procedures help to rationalize decision making.

Decision making is an important skill in helping service practice as well as in everyday life. Practitioners can help their clients decide courses of action through the use of decision-making procedures, thereby enhancing their client's problem-solving growth. Using such techniques for decision making in administrative practice and in selecting solutions for the development of new helping service technology (procedures, programs and policy) rationalizes a process that frequently is given little attention in the total problem-solving process.

ADDITIONAL READINGS

Andre L. Delbecq, Andrew H. Van de Ven and David H. Gustafson. *Group Techniques for Program Planning: A Guide to Nominal Group and Delphi Processes.* Glenview, IL: Scott, Foresman and Co., 1975.

Ronald W. Toseland, Robert F. Rivas and Dennis Chapman. "An Evaluation of Decision-Making in Task Groups," *Social Work*, Vol. 29, No. 4, July-August 1984, pp. 339-346.

C. H. Kepner and B. B. Tregoe. *The Rational Manager: A Systematic Approach to Problem Solving and Decision-Making.* New York: McGraw-Hill, 1965.

R. V. Brown, A. S. Kahr and C. Peterson. *Decision Analysis for the Manager.* New York: Holt, Rinehart and Winston, 1974.

EXERCISE – USING THE EVALUATION GRID FOR DIRECT PRACTICE

The evaluation grid can be a useful tool in any decision-making context. Use it by role playing a practitioner-client situation. For a designated problem ask the client to generate as many solutions as possible. Help the "client" sort the strategies from the ideas. Then encourage the client to produce broad criteria for evaluating them. Following this, help the client become more specific about each of the criteria produced. Determine mutually those criteria that are most important for selecting a strategy. Using a simple rating system, e.g., good, fair, poor, ask the client to rate the strategies on the criteria chosen. Discuss the results with the "client." What are the results? Does the "client" believe that this strategy will be effective? Can it be implemented?

Following this discussion, "practitioner" and "client" should tell each other how they experienced their respective roles. How did the decision-making process work? Are their other steps that need to be considered in it?

EXERCISE – PUTTING IT ALL TOGETHER

This exercise will *test* your understanding of the chapter material and, as well, will *expand* your understanding of it. It is a group exercise. Moving through the various steps of solution finding is an excellent way to recognize how the subjective and objective merge in an evaluation process. The group should allow itself two hours for this exercise.

Convene a group of four to six members who have recently produced a large number of solutions for solving a problem. The group's task is to find the solution or solution package that, in its judgment, best solves the problem. These are the following steps the group should take:

1. Classify solutions by identifying strategies or ideas. Identify in both groups those that are similar in content. Clarify whether there are redundancies in these groups. Eliminate those solutions that are redundant.
2. Produce as many broad criteria for evaluating the strategies as possible. Remember to defer judgment while doing so.
3. Again, deferring judgment generate criteria-spurring questions to each of the broad criteria produced in step 2.
4. Transform each question produced in step 3 into conceptual form. Try for simplicity of expression.
5. Decide through group discussion which criteria are most important for evaluating the strategies. Choose as many as five, but no fewer than three criteria. Full group participation in this step is crucial for the total decision-making process.
6. Weight each criterion by using the method of paired-comparison. Rely on thorough group discussion when making comparisons between criteria and determining the weightings.
7. Decide upon a scale for rating each solution relative to the criteria. Rate each solution on every criterion. Full discussion of the group should precede the actual selection of a rating. Multiply the weighting of each criterion by the rating given each solution. Find the numerical total for each solution by adding all solution-criterion boxes within the evaluation grid.

8. Compare the numerical ratings for the solutions. What do the
   results suggest? Do the numerical results make good sense?
   What decisions follow from this evaluation procedure? Is there
   any way of combining solutions that have nearly equivalent
   ratings into a *solution package*? What should be done with
   solutions that were not rated highly but may have potential for
   the future?
9. If time allows repeat the above procedure by first generating
   ideas to the strategies chosen and then moving through the rest
   of the decision-making steps.

Chapter 9

Acceptance Finding: Planning and Acting

Acceptance finding, the last stage of the CPS process, has as its goals the planning, implementation and evaluation of the solution selected in the solution-finding stage.

Planning as used in the acceptance-finding stage of CPS does not have as broad a meaning as planning definitions often found in the helping service literature. For example, Gilbert and Specht define planning as "the conscious attempt to solve problems and control the course of future events by foresight, systematic thinking, investigation, and the exercise of value preferences in choosing among alternative lines of action" (1977, p. 1).

As can be seen, this definition includes such problem-solving activities as finding alternatives for solution, decision making and acceptance finding. This definition of planning is too broad for our purposes. Dror, from the field of public administration, defines planning more inclusively: he says planning is "the process of preparing a set of decisions for action in the future directed at achieving goals by optimal means"(1964). This definition most closely fits with what planning means in the acceptance-finding stage of CPS (Figure 42).

York (1982) has identified a number of important factors that are associated with planning activities. They are as follows:

1. Planning is *future-oriented*. It is an attempt to implement today's decisions tomorrow.
2. Planning is a *continuous process*. Although it is conceivable that a planner or planning group may develop a plan of action

in one meeting that reaches the intended objectives this result is highly unlikely. Planning is an ideal process. It is a conception of how we want things to work. And the world, all too frequently, meets our planning efforts with, at best, relative indifference and, at worst, with resistance. Plans must be frequently changed. Therefore, planning is an ongoing, continuous process that requires adaptability, flexibility and creativity.

3. Planning and decision making are *inextricably related*. The plans that we make must clearly correspond to the decisions made earlier. Planners can lose sight of these decisions with the result that a plan cannot meet the desired objective implied in the selected solution.

4. Planning relates *means to ends*. Essentially the means for reaching the planning goal are sub-goals. Each of these sub-goals must contribute to the desired end. The planner or planning team must be aware that there are alternative ways to reach sub-goals (means) and that the choice among them must be made based upon its ability to optimally contribute to the goal.

Planning, therefore, is a future-oriented, continuous process, inextricably related to decision making which attempts to convincingly relate means to ends.

ADVANTAGES OF PLANNING

What are the advantages of planning? First, planning, although it cannot guarantee a certain future, makes the actions that must be taken to reach the goal *specific*. Planning decreases uncertainty. In addition, planning for implementing a creative solution helps establish *long- and short-term goals* for the individual workers and work groups, thereby helping them gain a sense of accomplishment when these goals are reached (Bricker & Cope, 1977, p. 9). Thirdly, planning helps those involved in the process to recognize the *coordination* that is necessary if any meaningful goal is to be reached. Because most helping service solutions involve not only client and worker the intended goal can likely include coordination between a large set of actors. Specialization within the helping services has

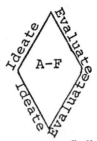

FIGURE 42. The acceptance-finding stage of CPS.

made coordination between social agencies difficult. Development of new programs for the delivery of services may involve the interrelationship between a whole range of specialized resources. For example, the planning of a new service for seniors may involve coordination with nurses, doctors, physical and recreational therapists, architects, social workers, etc.

Finally, planning encourages *accountability*. The goal you, either individually or with your planning team, wish to reach must not only be creative, it must also have a rational plan for backing it. This kind of plan provides the constituency and major decision makers who hold the power to approve or veto the project a better understanding of the project and how it can meet the social need for which it is intended. A coherent plan gives the individual or group client system the confidence and the motivation to continue the arduous work of implementing it in treatment and in the outside world.

PLANNING LIMITATIONS

Planning is limited by the quality invested in the process. Planning involves the use of skills and techniques that aid the planning process. Without such skills and methods, planning will be poor. Good planning input is necessary for good results when the plan is made operative. As analogy, consider the computer. If faulty data is fed into a computer it is clear that the output from the computer will be ineffective for making good decisions. As the saying goes — garbage in, garbage out.

Even though planning is sound and skillful in execution a plan may fail because the plan is never put into operation. Planners must believe in the plan and be committed to action for the plan to succeed. Belief in the planning process comes from the experience of working through a carefully thought-out plan and reaching some measure of success. If some members of a planning team perceive planning as an "academic exercise" it is best to identify those members who are strongly committed to the plan and who wish to be the implementors of action. It is only through an action orientation that the solution changes from an idea to a concrete reality.

PLANNING TECHNIQUES

Planning is usually characterized as a systematic, highly rational and analytical process. I believe it is so considered because the end result appears to the observer not involved in planning as a process that follows from the goal in a *logical* manner. In *part* planning *is* a logical process. But in keeping with the CPS process it can make use of imaginative operations of the mind to make it an integrated process. Remember that Gilbert and Specht defined planning as including the element of *foresight*. Translated into creative terms foresight is basically the ability to visualize future possibilities and probabilities. The person who, colloquially, has vision is one who is able to *see* into the future and to recognize new directions to take. Planning, then, requires a blend of imaginative and logical techniques. The techniques that I am going to suggest as tools for aiding the planning process, i.e., the 3M technique and checklisting, all involve this blend between the imaginative and the logical.

The 3M Technique

The Mini-Mental Movie (3M) is a planning technique that depends upon visualizing each step required to gain the plan's acceptance, to accomplish and insure its effectiveness and evaluate the chosen solution or solution package. It is highly effective when used by a group, for in group the number of ideas gained through visualization is greater than when employed alone. Below are sequential steps used in the 3M technique:

1. A planning group of four to five members is convened. Not all members of the group necessarily must be involved with the total CPS process. In fact, there are benefits for including persons who have not been involved with the process, particularly when the group has not had prior experience in planning.

2. The group members, on an individual basis, visualize each planning step as best they can, from the beginning of the implementation of the solution to its end. Members are asked "what would be the first step you would take in getting this step implemented? How would you accomplish it? What are the next steps? How would you gain acceptance for the idea? Include gaining acceptance activities in your visualizations. Remember also to include steps for measuring the effectiveness of your solution once it is implemented. Try to be as complete as possible in your visualizations. As you visualize a step write it down on paper. Or, if this bothers you, write down all your steps after the time is up." How much time should be given for this step? Through experience I have found that the time should expand with the amount of planning experience and visualizing ability of the group members. A group with little or no planning experience may finish their visualizing in five to ten minutes. Lack of visualizing skill may also shorten the time required in this step, although with a group leader's support members may be motivated to "see" more deeply into what is necessary for a good plan. This step is completed when all group members have written on paper all steps they believe are necessary for the implementation of the idea.

3. All steps are shared in the group. Each member either reads out their list of steps or, if possible, places them on chart paper or a chalkboard so all members can view them. Group members then identify duplicate steps and eliminate one of them from the lists. Steps that are apparently the same must be discussed to discern whether differences between them do exist and both should be kept. Any steps that are not understood by group members should be clarified.

4. Following the sharing, clarification and elimination of duplicate planning steps group members must *converge* upon those

steps believed to be most significant for inclusion in the plan. This requires involved discussion and participation by all members. The culmination of this process is the selection and *sequential ordering* of all necessary planning steps.

5. The group members must defer judgment in this step. For each step in the planning sequence they must produce who? what? where? why? why? and how? questions. Consider, for example, a group that is working out a plan to implement the idea of producing a crime prevention kit for public education. The group members diverge by asking questions related to the step of distributing the kit. Where should it be distributed? Who should distribute it? When will the kit be ready for distribution? What reaction or response do we want from those accepting the kit? From those rejecting it? What form of distribution best favors acceptance of the kit? Why should distribution of the kit be the responsibility of the planning group? Who else might distribute it? How can we persuade another group to accept the distribution task? As can be seen each question that is framed, requires an answer, and these answers, found through investigation and research, form the sub-steps of the plan. (See Table 2 for an example of a plan that has been completed using this questioning technique.)

6. When the group has generated questions to each of the ordered steps in the plan the group must then assign to individual members the tasks of finding information to answer some of them. Not all questions that have been produced will require information. Some of the questions require that the group produce alternative ideas to the question and then select *that* alternative that best serves the plan. For example, in Step #5 above, a group member asked the question: *Where should the kit be distributed?* This question makes necessary the generation of ideas from the planning group about physical location of distribution. The ideas that the group generates may then lead to an investigation of these various locations to determine the best one. Alternatively, the question *what reaction or response do we want from those accepting the kit?* may require some answers that come readily to the group and then lead to another planning sub-step. If the group wants formal response from

TABLE 2

STEPS	WHO	WHAT	WHERE	WHEN	WHY	HOW
#1 Read literature and discuss with experts in order to get information on problem in general, and on work already been done with young victims of racism.	Talk to social worker at community center in multi-racial setting.	Discuss social worker's experiences dealing with kids with negative self identities.	Arrange to meet worker at place of work. Might be good to talk to him in his work setting.	Decide time & duration of interview. Also set convenient date	In order to get first-hand understanding of problem in general and how expert sees it.	Do research before interview so to design relevant questions and propose important issues.
#2 Obtain knowledge and understanding of problem in own work context, and on work being done to counter-act it there.	Talk to own co-workers and clients and other important people at agency.	Discuss the nature and scope of the problem in agency setting setting	At agency - in both formal and informal meetings. Also in community.	At pre-set times and at unscheduled times. On an on-going basis.	To become more aware of problem as it relates to agency context.	After initial feedback devise questions and other means of obtaining appropriate information.
#3 Begin to make nature and scope of problem known within agency and suggest need for intense problem-solving effort on the part of workers.	Talk to co-workers at agency ensuring that all are made aware of problem.	Elaborate on enormity of problem and suggest ways of alleviating it in own agency setting.	Begin to talk about this at staff meeting or call special meeting.	Call a special meeting at a time when people are not pushed or under pressure so they have time	To seek co-worker feedback and insight into their understanding and interest in problem.	Send around memo asking staff to attend meeting briefly outlining purpose of this gathering.
#4 utilize any others of staff support and actively seek out their understandings of problem and what should be done to eradicate it. Encourage staff involvement.	Seek out workers who are likely to be facing this problem in their day-to-day work.	Ask them to support you and to help design new ways of dealing with problem.	Obtain info within agency and in community.	Set specific meeting time(s) to talk about ideas and discuss on informal basis	In order to get new ideas and fresh outlook on problem.	Spark their interest in idea of a treatment kit showing how they might use it with clients to enhance work.

TABLE 2 (continued)

STEPS	WHO	WHAT	WHERE	WHEN	WHY	HOW
#5 Before worker(s) begin to put together treatment kit they must first have an awareness of own values, those of agency and profession and how these might affect work.	Look to own selves as well as co-workers to gain insight and value awareness.	Be aware of positive and negative attitudes and how they might affect their ability to work at agency.	Observe behaviour at agency with clients and in community	Observe on on-going basis and then hold seminar to help gain awareness of feelings.	In order that treatment kit designed later will be effective and not be subject to any biases.	Design different value-Clarification tasks for workers to assess their biases which might influence work.
#6 Important for workers to know needs of particular racial clientele and what these clients themselves perceive to be their needs.	Talk to ethnic clients who use services and those who are likely to do so in future.	Find out the cultural heritage of group(s) and what their racial identity means to them.	Talk to clients at the agency and in community setting.	On an on-going basis and on certain dates	To gain a real understanding of how clients see problem affecting them.	Set up client-worker task-force for purpose of gathering data.
#7 Design treatment kit. Include worker goals, preparatory and beginning work, and client-worker tasks. Also use analogy to explain helping relationship.	Utilize a variety of resources--co-workers, clients, and other experts.	Treatment kit will be designed to provide no. of techniques for workers counseling young victims.	The kit will be assembled at the agency.	Specific dates will be set aside to work on kit.	Kit will be vital in helping workers enable client to work on feelings of racial inferiority.	work designing of kit around resources -- staff, money, information, equipment, to ensure its quality.
#8 Be attuned to specifics in the kit and plan for these on a separate basis. This is to ensure efficiency and effectiveness on an individual basis.	Look to co-workers with special skills to help plan and carry these out.	Individual plans will include such tasks as putting together a slide show.	Slides will be taken in surrounding multi-racial community.	Slides will be taken on set date(s) and then will be assembled by workers.	The purpose of the slide show will be to enable client to see good aspects of racial groups.	Again resources will have to be utilized in a constructive and profitable way.

TABLE 2 (continued)

STEPS	WHO	WHAT	WHERE	WHEN	WHY	HOW
#9 Once the treatment kit is put together then the worker(s) must get their agency to see worthiness of kit and to back them in their search for funding.	Look within agency to interested co-workers and recruit their effort to persuade reluctant ones.	Sell idea of treatment kit as effective aid for workers, and help them see need for $ to implement.	First, must gather the support of agency co-workers and community before going to outside sources.	Advocate on behalf of kit on an on-going basis and call special meeting to promote it at agency.	Want to get support of agency so that they will help influence funders in order to get money.	Send preliminary draft of kit to co-workers and then call a meeting to discuss this. Allow for worker input.
#10 Pressure a no. of outside sources for necessary funding. Can look to both the private and public sector for monies.	All three levels of government, private donors, foundations and other sources can be focused on.	Draw up effective presentation of treatment kit – portraying need and creative solution.	Give presentations in own community, as well as at places of convenience for target funding	Arrange set dates and times in order to present kit to various target funding sources.	Purpose of getting $ will be to allow for implementation of kit and to ensure it's quality.	Draw up introductory letters and send to target pop. Follow up with phone calls to arrange specific meet. Indicates.
#11 Implement kit on trial basis. Have on-going assessment and evaluation providing for client and worker feedback as part of this process.	Look to those workers and clients who have already begun to use the kit in their help-ing process.	Evaluate the total kit and try to gain new ideas from those using kit, so to make it more effective.	Do this on an informal basis and also design workshop where an in-depth assessment of kit can evolve/	Set aside times to meet with workers and clients on an individual basis and plan date for workshop	Purpose of this procedure will be to improve the kit so that it will better enable workers to help	Evaluate on short-term basis only. Always encourage on-going evaluation on part of workers and clients
#12 Monitor relative success of kit and alter it in light of feedback. Then report findings and changes to agency funders and signifi-cant others.	Report to workers in agency, funders, other agencies interested in this problem and interested others.	Relate the negative and positive aspects of kit focusing on the positive and showing constructive changes	At own agency in community at work places of funders and other relevant agencies if interested.	Again set aside certain dates and times in order to report findings.	to prove the legitimacy of the kit and ensure continued support both within and without agencies.	Design different ways and means of reliably portraying accurate and adequate information.

those accepting the kit, a short questionnaire must then be made and tested for effectiveness. Step #6 is completed when all questions have been answered through the generation of ideas and research and investigation.

7. The plan is now complete. A thorough review of it in its completed state should now be undertaken. Such questions as the following should be considered: what step(s) of the plan appear less strong than the others? Is there anything we might do to strengthen them? Is the plan clear, concrete and specific? Does each sub-step in the plan have a date for completion? Are the times that have been allocated to complete a sub-step realistic? Should more time be allocated for certain sub-steps? Is the plan completely ready to be put into action?

8. The plan upon completion of the review is put into operation.

The 3M technique is a comprehensive approach to the task of developing a concrete and clear plan for action. However, a final plan cannot guarantee its success. A plan is never final and as the plan moves from the drawing board into the real world of action it is bound to be modified. For example, my plan to make a videotape of the CPS process included five actual shooting sessions, one to tape the learning session, three sessions for taping the various stages of the process and one participant reaction session. An additional taping session was necessary because of technical problems. It may be obvious to many that plans frequently require change as they are implemented. There is no harm in being prepared mentally for these changes. The good planner must have the capacity to be flexible and adaptable as the plan becomes action. The action comes up against the fantasies and foresight of the planner and tests not only the planner's adequacy in this regard but action also causes reaction. No matter how carefully prepared a plan may be, particularly in regard to the steps planners have taken to gain its acceptance by decision-makers and other influential persons, a plan's action engages the individuals it effects on various levels of awareness. Intellectually, the plan may be readily accepted by those it touches; on the emotional level it may breed negative feelings that have to be accommodated through *political* acumen. Therefore, a plan as it confronts the individual actors that it must engage can become a series of careful negotiations. As York has noted in regard to the use of planning technology:

> . . . it is acknowledged that although the employment of this [planning] technology will enhance the probability of a rational decision outcome, it will surely not guarantee it. Political considerations will often carry greater weight in the determination of human service decisions. (1982, p. 204)

The creative problem solver, whether involved in the development of an individual treatment plan or a highly complex design of a service project must be aware of the political implications of the plan.[1]

Exercise — Using the 3M Technique

This exercise will provide practice in the use of the 3M technique. Convene a group of four to five persons. Use a solution that requires a plan for implementation. Follow each of the eight steps of the 3M technique. Attempt to produce a plan that has as many as eight sequential steps, with four to five sub-steps included in each of the major steps.

Set aside at least two hours for this exercise. Present your finished plan to another group and encourage their feedback to the plan. On the whole would they accept it or reject it? If they would reject it can they identify the major parts of it that need reworking? If so, spend some time attempting to rework these areas of the plan.

The Checklisting Technique

Noller, Parnes and Biondi (1977) have developed a list of thirty questions that serves as a checklist in the implementation of a plan to reach a creative solution (see Table 3). The questions are employed as part of a procedure that is called the checklisting technique. This technique, as does the 3M planning technique, calls for

---

[1]As this topic goes beyond the scope of this book, the reader is referred to Brager and Hollaway for an excellent discussion of the politics of change. See George Brager and Stephen Hollaway, *Changing Human Service Organizations: Politics and Practice* (New York: The Free Press, 1978).

both divergent and convergent thinking. The technique requires the following steps:

1. Quickly move through the list of questions and write down your immediate response to as many of them as you can. If you cannot answer a question move on to the next one.
2. Go through the list of questions again. This time turn each question around, upside down or sideways in an attempt to get different responses to them. These responses may lead to different perspectives and insights that may help in planning. For example, consider question 13: who might help with the idea? This question might be turned into—who might not help with the idea? or who might be helped if they help with the idea? or, who, if they help with the idea, might improve it? Try to answer these questions as best you can. The object of this step is to think divergently so many alternative ways of viewing the question's central theme can be generated.
3. Next, identify those questions that you have been unable to answer. Ask yourself: are any of those questions crucial for planning your solution? If so, you must research and investigate to get answers for them. If this procedure is carried out in a group assign various members to research answers to critical questions.
4. When you no longer are able to produce answers to the checklist look over your answers, determine those that best lead to a sound action plan and then construct the plan.

An Illustration of the Checklisting Procedure

Following is an example of a partial use of the checklisting technique for planning. Four questions have been chosen for the illustration: 1, 7, 17 and 20. The problem that requires solution is—how can our training and staff development department improve the effectiveness of new child protection workers. The solution selected for implementation is the development of a training laboratory that stimulates the many problem situations faced by protective workers.

QUESTIONS

1. What might I do to gain acceptance? How? When? Where? Why?
2. What might I do to gain enthusiasm for the idea? How? When? Where? Why?
3. What might I do to insure effectiveness? How? When? Where? Why?
4. What ways might I use criteria to show advantages? How might I demonstrate or dramatize this? Where? When? Why?
5. What other advantages might there be? How might I dramatize these? When? Where? Why?
6. What disadvantages might there be? How might I overcome these? When? Where? Why?
7. What additional resources might help (individual, groups, money, materials, equipment, time, authority, permission, other intangibles, etc.)? How might I obtain them? When? Where? Why?
8. What new challenges might the idea suggest?
9. How might I anticipate and meet these? When? Where? Why?
10. What objections, difficulties, limitations, obstacles might there be?
11. How might I overcome them? When? Where? Why?
12. How might I improve, safeguard, or fortify the idea? When? Where? Why?
13. Who might help with the idea? How? When? Where? Why?
14. What group might help? How? When? Where? Why?
15. Who might contribute special strengths or resources? How? When? Where? Why? How might I get them to help? When? Where? Why?
16. Who might add an unexpected element? How? When? Where? Why?
17. Who might gain from the idea? How? When? Where? Why?
18. Who might need persuasion? How? When? Where? Why?
19. How might I reward myself or others for helping carry out the idea? When? Where? Why?
20. How might I pretest my idea? When? Where? Why?
21. What first steps might I take to initiate action? How? When? Where? Why?
22. What next steps might follow? How? When? Where? Why?
23. What timing might I use? How/ When? Where? Why?
24. What schedules might I follow? How? When? Where? Why?
25. What follow-up to provide feedback to measure the progress? How? When? Where? Why?
26. What follow-up to allow corrective measures? How? When? Where? Why?
27. What follow-up to deal with unexpected repercussions? How? When? Where? Why?
28. What special times might I use? Days? Dates? How? Where? When? Why?
29. What special circumstances or occasions might I use? How? When? Where? Why?
30. What special places or locations might I use? How? When? Where? Why?

TABLE 3. Thirty Question Checklist. Ruth B. Noller, Sidney J. Parnes, and Angelo M. Biondi, excerpted from *Creative Actionbook*. Copyright © 1976, Charles Scribner's Sons. Reprinted with the permission of Charles Scribner's Sons.

QUESTION	ANSWER
1. What might I do to gain acceptance?	Talk with training director; encourage all planning members to be enthusiastic about the solution: talk to protection workers about solution; talk with Director of Protection Services about idea; talk with Agency Director.
How?	Set up meetings with each of the above.
When?	Preferably in the morning when they are fresh; make sure they have plenty of time to chat about idea; meet at their convenience.
Where?	Meet on their turf; talk about idea with protection workers informally over coffee, lunch.
Why?	To gain support for idea; get feedback for idea — does it need more input?

DIVERGING QUESTIONS	ANSWERS
1. What might I not do to gain acceptance?	Make sure I present idea as accomplished fact; oversell idea; be too brash and aggressive when talking with decision-makers; schedule meetings at my convenience; have meetings right after lunch, discourage other planning members from discussing idea with fellow workers.
What might I do to accept our solution?	Know exactly the methods required to make it work; agree that these methods are good ones; immerse myself in training literature on simulations; recognize the solution's limitations and attempt to find solutions for them.

QUESTION	ANSWERS
What additional resources might help (individuals, groups, money, materials, equipment, time, authority, permission, other intangibles, etc.)?	Training professional's expertise; information from protection workers; information from business and industry training departments that have simulated programs; can grants be obtained? Do professional helping service organizations have information? Can we get electronic equipment donated from various companies as public relations gestures.
How?	Write and call various organizations; set up appointments for interviews when appropriate.

DIVERGING QUESTIONS	ANSWERS
What additional resources might hinder?	Too much material from established training programs might influence us in their direction; conventional opinion of some trainers might dissuade us from our solution; funding from federal and state sources might require slanting the training program toward their interests.
What additional resources might encourage others to help?	If we find some funding outside of agency, decision-makers within the agency might be strongly amenable to solution; recommendations from outside sources may influence inside decision-makers.
Who might gain from the idea?	Protection workers; clients helping service professions; the total agency; children; Training and Staff Development Department; social invention team; funders; Agency Director.

How?

Better training should lead to more effective service and better client benefits; new training methods could be diffused within child welfare field; training methods may have effects on other kinds of training methodology; if training is successful agency will be considered an innovator and get publicity; funders get prestige.

DIVERGING QUESTIONS

ANSWERS

Who might not gain from the idea?

Everyone mentioned above; idea might fail; research might show that standard training procedure is just as effective.

What gain might accrue if idea failed?

Training Department might learn how to improve training from its mistakes; feedback from trainees might help invention team develop better training methods; evaluation procedures might look at methodological and theoretical training issues and identify important conceptual problems for training that go beyond immediate training situation.

Who might lose the most from idea?

The social invention team; clients and workers.

How might I pretest my idea?

Train small sample of workers and compare with standard training group.

When?

Three months before actual project is to start.

Where?

Within agency setting.

Why?

To determine changes needed in training program; to get feedback from trainees.

DIVERGENT QUESTIONS	ANSWERS
How might I not pretest my idea?	Do nothing; assume training program is ready to go as planned; be arrogant, overconfident.
How might I pretest idea without using protective workers?	Use helping service workers from other units in agency; use non-professionals for the pretest; recruit students for the training.

As can be seen the process of attempting to answer the checklist questions and, as well, to generate other questions about them can lead to a huge quantity of information. This information is the data bank used to make a concrete and thorough plan. The plan is made by transforming these data into a step-by-step guide for implementing and evaluating the effects of the intended solution. The checklisting procedure is a helpful tool for producing the information necessary for constructing a working plan. The data is generated by divergent and convergent means and then convergently selected for use in the plan based upon judgments made upon their importance.

IMPLEMENTATION

Once the plan is complete we must move toward its implementation. In the case of the human service worker who is working with an individual, group or family unit there is little question that it is both the client system and the worker who must be involved in the implementation of the plan. The worker must intervene in this stage when contacts outside of the client system must be influenced. But who is required to act when we are attempting to implement a new program or project? If we have a planning team involved, as is often the case, who among these members becomes the actors? These questions are important because there may exist differing learning styles among the planners leading to a differing program or project interests.

Kolb et al. (1974) have classified learning styles in four categories. In Figure 43 we see that there is an ideal learning cycle. The effective learner reflects upon concrete experiences, develops abstractions based upon this reflection and then tests out these new concepts in life situations. It has been noted, however, that this cycle may be difficult for many to complete.

> [S]ince the learning process is directed by individual needs and goals, learning styles become highly individual in both direction and process. For example, a mathematician may come to place great emphasis on abstract concepts, whereas a poet may value concrete experience more highly. A manager may be primarily concerned with active application of concepts, whereas a naturalist may develop his observational skills highly. Each of us in a more personal way develops a learning style that has some weak points and strong points. We may jump into experiences but fail to observe the lessons to be derived from these experiences; we may form concepts but fail to test their validity. In some areas our objectives and needs may be clear guides to leaning; in others, we wander aimlessly. (1974, pp. 28-29)

Not only learning style is crucial in the implementation phase. The learning style appropriate to action must also be associated with the requisite skill. The implementation phase is one that requires not only action but action that is informed by reflection. The question that must be answered is how do we implement this action toward the desired outcome. Therefore action must be wedded to experience and wisdom for it to be effective.

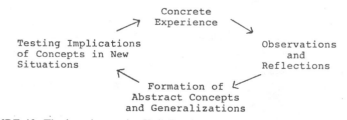

FIGURE 43. The learning cycle. Kolb/Rubin/McIntyre, *Organizational Psychology: An Experiential Approach*, © 1974, p. 28. Reprinted by permission of Prentice-Hall, Inc., Englewood Cliffs, NJ.

Reducing Resistance to Change

A plan is a blueprint for change. Change, a neutral concept, can be threatening for many people. The implementor must employ a set of guidelines in the attempt to introduce change. Spedale (1972) has identified a number of such guidelines important in reducing resistance to change:

1. *Actively seek the maximum amount of co-participation* — help others in sharing ownership of the new idea and its plan. Don't hog ownership. Encourage everyone that will be affected by the plan to meaningfully feel a part of it.
2. *Become most sensitive to the change the plan contains* — when individuals' social interaction and interpersonal relations are changed they strongly resist, more so than if the procedures and methods by which they work are changed. Greater resistance occurs when they perceive themselves manipulated to change. To reduce this resistance fully inform those affected by the plan. Solicit their opinions about the proposed changes. If possible, invite their participation in the planning stage if feasible. Avoid confrontations while performing these tasks. Remember that the new information may threaten those most affected and can lead to anger. Understand the reason for this anger and attempt to help the people affected know you are concerned about their feelings about the planned change.
3. *Make clear how the plan provides something better for clients* — a pattern of working is not easily relinquished, no matter the level of its success. Individuals are reluctant to accept change unless they can see the benefits of it. Explore the social, psychological, economic and other benefits that can accrue from the implementation of the plan with those involved.
4. *Present the plan clearly and attractively* — frequently plans are not clearly understood when presented on a verbal level. A plan is an abstract design. Visual presentations of the plan using slides, transparencies or drawn diagrams help the person who is attempting to understand it to better comprehend

its various facets. Further, visuals demonstrate the planner's *interest* in helping others to understand the plan.

5. *Keep plan presentations simple* — whenever possible avoid technical language; jargon, acronyms and abbreviations frequently have mystifying consequences on your audience.

6. *Provide a complete picture of the plan* — providing the audience with only the positive aspects of an apparently new and exciting plan that has its devious side and can be seen as such. Present the probable negative aspects of the plan along with the ways in which the plan has incorporated ways of neutralizing these negative effects. Bringing the negative facets of a plan into the open before they are identified by the audience can produce trust in you and the plan.

7. *Present plans at an optimum time* — although an optimum time may vary with persons who are presented with a plan, a few guidelines should be kept in mind. Mornings are frequently better times to present than afternoons because more persons are alert between 9 to 11 than between 1 to 4. Make sure you have ample time to make the presentation. Know how much time you need and if you are asked to take less than the time required put off the meeting until more time can be afforded. Avoid presentations when you know your audience has such weighty matters as budgeting and reporting to do. Know when to best schedule meetings.

8. *Give credit for the idea and plan to others* — willingly share any credit that is given. Make sure you let others know that the project idea and plan was a collaborative effort.

9. *Share results of any pre-testing built into your plan* — such sharing lets interested parties know that you have a willingness to further develop and refine the plan. This feedback further involves individuals in the project.

10. *Be prepared to be flexible when presenting your plan* — the audience may be willing to offer support or other resources only if some modifications are made in the plan's implementation. The presenter should be open to new approaches to implementing the idea without necessarily agreeing to them. If a condition to receiving resources is such a plan change the

presenter must consult with team members and other key decision-making figures before an agreement is reached.

11. *When change can be adopted without approval, keep people informed* – a unit within a helping service agency may have the opportunity of planning and implementing change without gaining approval of those that will be affected. The innovation will have a greater chance of being looked upon favorably if: there is advisement that a change is being contemplated; the reasons and rationale for the change are given; the plan for implementation described in full; periodic progress reports regarding the change are made; and confirmation is given that the change is part of regular operations, asking that feedback is given on any observed problems due to the change.

Reducing resistance to change requires a two-pronged approach. Key decision-makers must be involved and influenced positively for the plan to go forward. Once the plan is accepted the implementors must regard with importance those persons most affected by the plan. The more opportunity for involvement that individuals most affected by the anticipated change have, the greater the probability will be that the change can be effectively implemented. All changes cannot be accompanied by maximum involvement of the persons affected by it; however, respect for the principle of involvement should make planners and implementors more sensitive to ways in which personnel can be creatively involved in planned change.

Summary

This chapter has discussed planning and its implementation in the acceptance-finding stage of the CPS process.

Planning has been defined as the process of preparing a set of decisions for future action which is directed at achieving goals by optimal means. Planning has been presented as a process that demands creativity, flexibility and adaptability. The techniques of the Mini-Mental Movie (3M) and Checklisting have been presented as approaches to creative and effective planning. These planning approaches can be used on an individual and small group basis.

The advantages of planning, i.e., making the plan specific; establishing short-term goals; emphasizing coordination; and encouraging accountability were discussed. Planning limitations — deficits in planning input and lack of planning commitment by the planners were noted.

Implementation has been viewed as the action flowing from the plan. Steps, or sub-goals in the plan, must be achieved for the problem solution to become a reality. There may be a necessity in distinguishing between planners and actors to make the plan's implementation effective. Learning styles may differ among the planning group. Those with a strong active orientation coupled with the ability to reflect carefully upon the consequences of such action are those members most suited to carry out plans.

Finally, a number of guidelines were presented for helping reduce resistance to innovation. Such factors as actively seeking coparticipation; becoming sensitive to the impact of the change upon others; and making clear how the plan changes things for client benefits were discussed.

ADDITIONAL READINGS

Robert Marsenich. "How to Teach the Steps of Change," *Training,* Vol. 20, No. 3, March, 1983, pp. 62-63.

Gordon L. Lippitt. *Visualizing Change: Model Building and the Change Process.* La Jolla, California: University Associates, 1973.

B. Googins, V. A. Capoccia and N. Kaufman. "The Interactional Dimension of Planning: A Framework for Practice," *Social Work,* Vol. 28, No. 4, July-August, 1983, pp. 273-277.

James G. March. "Footnotes to Organizational Change," *Administrative Science Quarterly,* Vol. 26, No. 4, December, 1981, pp. 563-577.

C. T. Kochler. "Project Planning and Management Technique." *Public Administration Review,* Vol. 43, No. 5, September-October, 1983, pp. 459-466.

Chapter 10

Monitoring and Evaluating the Solution

Intended solutions require evaluation. The CPS process incorporates evaluation research as a sub-stage in acceptance-finding, its planning, implementation and evaluation stage. The plan for the implementation of the solution should include ways in which to trial test the solution and, if necessary, to modify the solution in view of these results, and to conduct a full-scale evaluation research study of the problem solution (Figure 44).

Evaluation of social invention has been problematic in the helping services. Rivlin has addressed this problem of innovation evaluation (1970). She contrasts two approaches to innovation in the social services, health and education fields. *Random innovation*, she declares, describes a strategy in which various levels of system try new ways of providing social and health services without any attempt to determine their effectiveness or generalization to other locales and settings. This, Rivlin contends, was the state of affairs in the 1960s when many programs such as Headstart, Title I, and

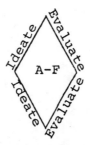

FIGURE 44. The acceptance-finding stage of CPS.

model cities were not designed to produce information on their effectiveness.

> The random innovation strategy of the 1960's produced tens of thousands of innovative projects. Some were wasteful or foolish; many simply increased the level of services delivered in much the same way; some were genuinely new and more effective. But most, including some of the more successful ones, never received national publicity. No one knows about them except the participants and the immediate community. Often they were unevaluated. The people who worked in them may have known they did a good job, but no visible or measurable statistics emerged that would convince someone else. (1970, p. 89)

Rivlin contrasts random innovation with *systematic experimentation*. She contends that innovations should be subject to scientific experimentation, with the innovation tried in enough places to establish its ability to be effective and the conditions in which it works most favorably. The innovation should be compared to other methods and/or with no methods or action at all. The innovation should be part of a *controlled* experiment.

In support of Rivlin's position is that of Fairweather (1967). He has declared that:

> The humanitarian approach to social problems *is* a research approach since its end goal is to separate those programs which provide the problems from those that are deleterious or not helpful. Social subsystems, whether designed for rehabilitation, education, aid to the socially disadvantaged, or whatever, can and should be subject to such experimentation. (p. 33)

There are, however, a number of reasons why it is difficult to carry out an ideal evaluation of social invention. Rothman, in his attempt to explain the relative lack of rigor in evaluating knowledge utilization and from it the development of practice tools, cites the *complexity* of the R&D process because it was involved with an intricitate social intervention (1980). Research methods and procedures were adapted to the R&D purpose rather than attempting to conform to conventional social science norms.

Patti has critiqued Rothman's ground breaking work in social R&D (1981). He states that Rothman should not have claimed success for the newly developed social technology issuing from the R&D effort because:

> The research methodology used in the main field test was essentially a pre-post test design without controls. . . . Given this methodology, there is any number of factors that might confound the relationship between the means (action guidelines) used and the outcomes obtained. (p. 42)

It is not only within the sphere of program evaluation that problems in research design occur. In recent years there has been a concerted effort to develop research designs for clinical helping service practice (Levy & Jayaratne, 1979). A problem within this development is identified by Nelsen (1981). She notes that:

> although most social workers are engaged in psychosocial treatment or use some combination of treatment models, most single-subject research to date has dealt with behavioral treatment. (p. 31)

The position that I take, however, is that if social invention is to be accepted on a scientific basis and hence more rapidly diffused and adopted, it must undergo rigorous experimental conditions. Until the invention can be associated with results that can convince helping service professionals of its effectiveness the invention must only be considered as provocatively interesting but without substantial usefulness to the profession.

MONITORING AND EVALUATING SOCIAL INVENTIONS

Monitoring

Monitoring is the process in which information about an inventive intervention is produced and analyzed. *Treatment monitoring* is an attempt to determine whether a client is receiving the intended intervention that is consistent with prior treatment planning, professional values and standards and the contract between the client and the worker (Tripodi & Epstein, 1980). As a hypothetical example consider the helping service worker who has developed an invention for helping couples reduce conflict. The invention is simple: one or both partners must stop talking to one another for at least fifteen minutes when conflict is recognized. To monitor the intervention the helping service worker prepares forms that the partners must fill out regarding their conflict behavior on a daily basis. The helping service worker wants to know if the couple is carrying out the intervention as planned and contracted. Further monitoring occurs when the helping service worker meets weekly with the couple and discusses any difficulties in employing the intervention.

Treatment Monitoring

Treatment monitoring as a total process includes these steps:

1. *Setting treatment standards*, e.g., workers should offer high levels of emotional support to recently released mental patients; workers who have five years of practice experience or more should deliver higher levels of empathic understanding than workers who have less than two years' experience; treatment given by newly graduated helping service workers should be supervised on a week-to-week basis;
2. *Generating, gathering and analyzing data concerning the attainment of these standards*, e.g., using forms, content analysis and data aggregation to determine if standards have been reached;
3. *Assessing discrepancies between planned and actual performance on the part of the worker and/or client*; and
4. *Deciding to continue, stop or change the intervention depending upon this assessment* (Tripodi & Epstein, 1980).

When employing a clinical invention for the first time it is crucial to monitor its use. Without systematic data it may be impossible to know whether the invention as planned is actually operating. Further, monitoring of a treatment invention may lead to its modification, such change making it more potent in effect. Feedback from the client at an early point in the invention's trial is a necessary part of the total social invention process, as well as a crucial part of any treatment intervention.

Program Monitoring

Program monitoring is an attempt to produce data for the periodic assessment of program activities. Questions that the monitoring process attempts to answer are: Is the program being carried out in accordance with the implementation plan? Is the targeted population for service being adequately served? Do the policies of the program and the activities that flow from them correspond and comply with the guidelines, laws and regulations that are imposed by professional bodies, external funding agencies and regulatory bodies?

These questions can be answered by employing such tools as surveys of the targeted client population being served; the use of forms to identify and clarify the activities of staff; and the use of sampling techniques for monitoring the performance of staff (Epstein & Tripodi, 1977).[1]

Program monitoring serves the same function for the program invention as does treatment monitoring for the treatment invention. It serves to determine whether the activities actually planned are operating and working as intended. Discrepancies between plan and its operation can be corrected. Changes in the program operation can be corrected. Changes in the program operation can be made to fit the reality of the service situation.

Evaluation

Evaluation, as is true for monitoring, can be classified according to *treatment* and *program*.

Treatment evaluation emphasizes the effectiveness and effi-

---

[1]An excellent treatment of both treatment and program monitoring for students and helping service practitioners, without a high level of research sophistication, has been made by Epstein and Tripodi (1977) and Tripodi and Epstein (1980). Readers should consult these authors as well as the references at the end of the chapter as a complete treatment of these topics is beyond the scope of this book.

ciency of one helper with one client system, either individual, family, or group. By *effectiveness* is meant the validity that a particular intervention has upon a problem—whether a problem is reduced or resolved by a particular action. By *efficiency* is meant the cost in time, money and manpower to effect change. A treatment intervention may be effective in the long run but highly inefficient. An example of such a treatment procedure is psychoanalysis which may reduce neurotic suffering in the distant future but certainly, because of the many years it requires, the amount of money expended by the client and the time expended by the analyst, cannot be considered efficient.

Program evaluation is an attempt to scrutinize the effectiveness and efficiency of total programs within an agency setting. For example, consider the child welfare agency that attempts to determine whether its adoption program has been successful in matching children and parents and whether the program's expenditures justify its efforts.

Treatment and program evaluation correspond when results from the work of more than one helper and the treatment outcomes from more than one client system are aggregated. Think of the treatment invention whereby the reduction of conflict is attempted by withdrawal of one or both partners. If a social agency engaged all of its family treatment unit in such an attempt, whereby eight couples were treated in exactly the same way (same treatment strategy) for the purpose of reaching the same treatment objectives, i.e., the reduction of conflict, we have an example of the correspondence between treatment and program evaluation.

BASIC DESIGNS FOR TREATMENT AND PROGRAM EVALUATION

Treatment Evaluation

There are various approaches to the evaluation of a treatment invention. One approach is to *survey* the client or clientele served by the specific intervention. In this way data are gathered that may help us understand the way treatment was perceived by clients, what use was made of the treatment intervention and whether clients served believed they received any lasting benefits. Unfortunately, an evaluation that counts upon survey data gathered after treatment, although it may shed light on the process and outcome of treatment, has little scientific standing if our goal is to attempt a linkage between invention and treatment outcome.

There are many factors that might intervene in the treatment process to confound the results and the survey approach to evaluation cannot account for them. Campbell and Stanley (1963) have identified a number of factors that can contaminate the validity of uncontrolled research findings. For example, *maturational factors* may be operating while the treatment is taking place; the *selection* of the sample of clients may be biased; *unusual events* may occur to the client during the treatment process, say a sudden gain in occupational success or a death in the family; and clients chosen for study may *leave treatment* in high numbers, leading to false generalizations founded upon those clients that remain.

These, and other factors, may be operative when evaluation is based upon a *pretest-posttest evaluation* design. The model for this design is shown in Figure 45 where X represents measurement and T indicates treatment.

Factors that can be added to the list above for confounding uncontrolled evaluation such as the pretest-posttest design are: *client reactions* to measurement; *faulty measurement tools*, i.e., those not standardized, therefore not reliable; *statistical regression*, the tendency of those chosen for the study based upon some extreme measurement score to subsequently regress to a more average score; and *interaction effects*, the possibility that all factors that Campbell and Stanley have identified may combine to produce a false conclusion to the evaluation study.

The Interrupted Time-Series Design

The interrupted time-series design, while it cannot control for all the factors that have been identified as possibly confounding study results, does give the invention evaluator the benefit of generating data prior to, during and after the intervention. What this means is that the evaluator is able to establish a *baseline* prior to treatment so later comparisons can be made with it. Such comparisons may then

$$X_1 \quad T \quad X_2$$

FIGURE 45. The pretest-posttest design.

reveal changes in behavior during and after treatment, therefore linking the treatment intervention with the observed change. As Tripodi and Epstein state:

> Although the interrupted time-series design does not control all factors affecting internal validity to which Campbell and Stanley referred, does not produce knowledge that is undisputably causal about the impact of treatment intervention, and does not produce findings that are immediately generalizable to other treatment cases, *this design can generate knowledge that is highly informative about the impact of treatment on a given client*. (1980, pp. 209-210)

Psychosocial Designs

Nelsen has raised the issue that single-subject research designs have concentrated upon behavioral objects such as smoking cessation, weight loss and improved school attendance even though most helping service workers practice within a psychosocial framework. She contends that single-subject evaluator's must learn to *target* intermediate goals rather than long-term final goals. The psychosocial practitioner, faced with intervening psychosocially with a woman who fears going outside because she is struggling to control her sexual feelings or anger, must develop a step-goal to measure rather than an end goal of complete freedom from these emotions as indicated by lack of fear of the external environment (Nelsen, 1981).

Nelsen divides intermediate treatment goals into *partial* and *instrumental* goals. She defines a *partial* goal "as a direct, recognizable step toward the achievement of a final goal." An example of a partial goal for our hypothetical women fighting with irrational sexual impulses might be a short walk to the mail box, a walk to the corner store or a brief shopping trip.

An *instrumental* goal is defined by Nelsen as "one that the practitioner or client assumes will lead toward a final goal by some indirect means, such as a change in the client's self-perception, or intrapsychic functioning." For example, a client who wishes to experience greater self-esteem may work with the helper toward increasing his assertiveness within his work team.

Nelsen's distinction between the end-goals of the behavioral practitioner and the partial and instrumental goals of the psychosocial practitioner is critical for many *treatment interventions* that may be of a psychosocial nature. They must be amenable to evaluation.

A PSYCHOSOCIAL TREATMENT INVENTION — A HYPOTHETICAL CASE

A young married couple experiencing conflict apply to a family agency for counseling. The husband, an unusually successful entrepreneur with a flair for a high-risk business ventures, claims his wife is frigid and is not interested in his hobbies, e.g., hiking, swimming and other active sports. The wife, on the other hand, an unusually attractive and soft-spoken young woman, contends that her husband does not understand her, is not subtle and does not know how to communicate on an intimate level.

Prior to the beginning of treatment the worker establishes that the husband does not *understand* the wife's friends or her parents. In conversation he frequently does not give empathic feedback and seldom gets the conversational point. The wife frequently does not kiss or touch her husband. With this information, the helper constructs instruments so that the couple can measure the frequency of these *partial* goals.

Treatment intervention begins with the worker serving as mediator to encourage the couple to discuss and explore their differences. After two sessions this intervention is recognized as hardening the positions of both the partners. The worker suggests a different approach — an invention — and the couple agree to it.

The invention is an attempt to construct dialogue about various problems that are presented. For example, this problem is presented to the couple — a father forbids his 16-year-old daughter to see a boy. What would be the viewpoint of the father, his wife, his daughter and the boy. Both partners are encouraged to say what each person in the scenario would think and feel. A variety of relatively ambiguous problems are given and the married couple share their reaction to each of the persons involved in the problems. Then they discuss their viewpoints and try to understand the reasons they may have for differences of opinion. These problems, viewpoint sharing and discussion are presented for three weeks. Following this three period a two week period ensued in which the couple's problems as initially presented are considered. For example – a successful married man feels dissatisfied because his wife seldom expresses interest in his activities. What would his viewpoint, his wife's and his and her friend's be to this situation. All viewpoints would be aired and discussed. Alternatively, a problem would be formulated like this: a married woman feels isolated because the husband spends nearly all of his time on his business and activities and doesn't share his feelings with her. What is his viewpoint, the wife's, her father's and mother's, his friend's, her friend's. Following these two weeks, the focus of the intervention shifted back to an exploration of the couple's difficulties in meeting each other's needs. Treatment ends after a twelve week period. Follow-up revealed relative success in reaching the global goals each partner established in the beginning of treatment.

Figures 46 and 47 illustrate hypothetical data for wife and husband on the partial goals that were established.

As can be seen, psychosocial treatment inventions can be evaluated, albeit imperfectly, with the interrupted time-series design. The practitioner must help clients clarify their partial or instrumental goals as steps toward the more global targets usually conceptualized in this type of treatment.

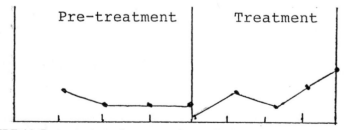

FIGURE 46. Pretreatment and treatment data on husband's partial goal of kissing and touching with wife (aggregated data).

Program Evaluation

Fairweather has developed methods for employing what he calls *Experimental Social Innovation* (1967, 1977).

Experimental Social Innovation calls for the selection of a social problem; the comparison of a program that represents an attempt to solve this problem with a program innovation; the careful attempt to equate both old and new programs through experimental means; the employment of the innovative program; collecting data on the effectiveness of old and new programs and drawing conclusions from analysis of this data.

Such an approach conforms with Rivlin's call for systematic experimentation. Fairweather's approach is a rigorous attempt to evaluate new social programs for the reduction of social problems. The design that Fairweather uses is a variation of the controlled experiment in that he uses a *comparison* group as a control. The paradigm for the controlled experiment is illustrated in Figure 48.

The controlled experiment as used for program evaluation has been specifically designed by Suchman (1967). He has identified three conditions that must be met for the design to be considered experimental.

The first condition is the existence of an equal chance for all subjects to be chosen for either the experimental or control group. *Random selection* must be used to draw the two groups from the population targeted for study. For example, if a social inventor de-

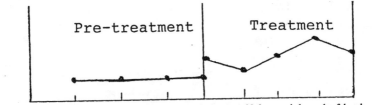

FIGURE 47. Pretreatment and treatment data on wife's partial goal of husband's improved listening behavior with wife's friends and parents (aggregated data).

X_1 T_1 X_2 - experimental group

X_1 T_2 X_2 - control group

FIGURE 48. The controlled experiment.

cides to study the effect of talking cessation on conflict reduction as a *program*, the inventor must identify a population of clients indicating conflict as their major problem and from this population, by random selection, compose a treatment and no treatment and/or comparison group. It should be recognized, however, that the population from which the groups are drawn define the degree to which the results of the experiment can be generalized. If, for example, we find that the treatment invention of withdrawal works for conflictful clients in the agency in which the study is taking place, we can only interpret our findings for this specific agency-related population.

Suchman identifies the careful specification of the program variables — the *independent variables* — as a second condition for the controlled experiment. Without such specification the study will not clarify what is producing the designed change or answer why the change is occurring. Consider a major attempt at program evaluation in social casework done in the 1960s (Meyer et al., 1965). The study, *Girls at Vocational High*, attempted to determine whether casework treatment given to an experimental group of delinquent girls was superior to a group not receiving help. The study demonstrated no differences between treatment and no-treatment groups. Why? Analysis of the research revealed that treatment was not clearly specified. Many different kinds of interventions were delivered under the rubric of social casework. Even if results had been obtained from this study, it would not have been possible to identify the *valid* treatment procedures.

Finally Suchman indicates a third required condition for the experimental method. The *dependent variable*, or the desired outcome of the experimental treatment, must be carefully defined and measured. As example, evaluating a program of talking cessation as a valid treatment procedure for conflict reduction must clearly specify what are considered indicators of this reduction.

CLASSIFYING PROGRAM EVALUATION

What should be evaluated in program evaluation? York (1982) has helped in answering this question by classifying evaluation according to the following seven criteria:

1. *Effort* — the evaluation attempts to determine the *quantity* of service provided or the *scope* of activities undertaken. For example, an agency attempts to learn how many clients it serves, the number of hours of client service it provides, and the different kinds of services it offers, etc.
2. *Efficiency* — efficiency is the evaluation criterion that relates the amount of resources, i.e., time, cost and manpower, to accomplishment. The question this type of evaluation attempts to answer is whether a service is cost-effective. Consider the experimental comparison of two day-care programs. The experimental program, it is found, requires fewer dollars to run and is equal in effectiveness to the control group. This program would then logically be the one selected for operation.
3. *Effectiveness* — to determine a program's effectiveness its achievements must be measured. The administration of a vocational rehabilitation program, for example, is interested in discovering how many of its clients receiving an innovative package of services are presently working as compared to a group that is receiving the regular kind of services. Did a new family treatment program produce such benefits as increased family cohesion, decreased parental-child conflict or increased parental self-esteem over a program that had been provided for years?
4. *Impact* — programs specify concrete indicators to evaluate their effectiveness. However, the programs may, in the long run, impact upon community-wide problems such as unemployment or juvenile delinquency. Although various programs may not have been designed to specifically address such problems, the combined effort of such programs, if scrutinized, may impress themselves upon the social problems in a geographical area.
5. *Quality* — quality refers to the evaluation of program standards such as the level of education and experience brought to bear upon program activities. The assumption in using these indicators of quality for evaluation is that high professional standards enhance program effectiveness. Helping service workers with masters degrees, it is assumed, will perform more effectively than workers who have undergraduate degrees. Although qual-

ity may lead to program effectiveness there is no hard evidence for such a relationship (Berman & Norton, 1985).

6. *Process* — a process evaluation is designed to determine what components of a program contributed to its success or failure. A number of program components can be identified: (a) the *attributes* of the program such as staff, method, program accessibility can clearly be related to a program's effectiveness; (b) the *population served* can have an effect on program success; (c) the *conditions* under which the program is offered can affect effectiveness. For example, one time of day may be most suitable for service delivery; paying for service as opposed to its being free may promote effectiveness; and (d) the *kind of effects* achieved by the program may or may not contribute to its effectiveness. For example, a program designed to improve the cognitive abilities of educationally retarded children may achieve attitudinal benefits instead.

7. *Equity* — when services are provided to a large population there is concern that such services are distributed fairly among the population. For example, an equity evaluation might attempt to determine whether unemployment benefits were delivered to all who are found eligible under the policies and procedures of such legislation. Such an evaluation should determine if practices are uniform from jurisdiction to jurisdiction and whether each is receiving its fair share of tax funds.

Evaluation research of program can be carried out along a number of different lines. The social inventor of programs must, however, be interested in the evaluation criteria of *effectiveness*, *efficiency* and *process* as those three that most significantly determine whether the social invention is worth continued application and diffusion and adoption by the social work profession.

Can Program Evaluation Be Done?

It may be strange to be confronted with the question whether program evaluation can be achieved after making a strong case for the necessity and importance of program evaluation if social invention is to be considered legitimate within the helping service field. Nevertheless, there are many obstacles that stand in the way of completing a controlled experiment.

First, it is often not possible to use random selection procedures to guarantee the equality of both experimental and control groups. Consider the evaluation of an educational program. Frequently program evaluators are forced to use a quasi-experimental design, wherein the comparison and/or control group is selected because it is convenient or *appears* similar in participant attributes, e.g., age, sex, educational status, experience, etc. Within the system in which the evaluation must be carried out are either educational, ethical, and administrative objections or a combination of all three that stand in the way of proceeding with random selection.

Further, the controlled experimental evaluation is expensive, requires a high level of cooperation among study participants, evaluator and administrative personnel. It may be ethically ruled out because it denies agency services to those in great service need.[2]

Summary

The CPS process has the ability to produce innovative solutions to micro- and macro-level problems, to problems that require the development of unique treatment procedures as well as to problems that demand creative program responses.

This chapter has emphasized the importance of research evaluation of both treatment and program invention. It has been shown that social innovation in the turbulent 1960s was characterized by *random innovation*, the lack of an attempt to garner systematic data about the effectiveness of the social innovation. After Rivlin and Fairweather, I have taken the position that rigorous research methods must be applied to social invention if invention is to be applied and diffused throughout the helping services.

Monitoring and evaluating, both of treatment and program, have

---

[2]For an excellent discussion of the various problems associated with steps in gaining approval for experimental program evaluation, the reader is referred to George Fairweather's *Methods of Experimental Social Innovation*, New York: John Wiley and Sons, 1967, Chapter 4.

been discussed. Examples of both processes have been presented.

The difficulties involved in rigorous treatment and program evaluation have not been minimized. As is true of all parts of the CPS process a flexible and creative response must be made to evaluation.

ADDITIONAL READINGS

Francis G. Caro (Ed.). *Readings in Evaluation Research*, 2nd ed. New York: Russell Sage Foundation, 1977.

Leonard Rutman (Ed.). *Evaluation Research Methods*. Beverly Hills, California: Sage Publications, 1977.

Jill Doner Kagle, "Evaluating Social Work Practice," *Social Work*, Vol. 24, No. 4, July, 1979, pp. 292-296.

Carl A. Bennett and Arthur A. Lumsdaine (Eds.). *Evaluation and Experiment: Some Critical Issues in Assessing Social Programs*. New York: Academic Press, 1975.

Carol H. Weiss, *Evaluation Research: Methods for Assessing Program Effectiveness*. Englewood Cliffs, N.J.: Prentice-Hall, 1972.

M. Hersen and D.H. Barlow. *Single-Case Experimental Designs: Strategies for Studying Behavior Change*. New York: Pergamon Press, 1976.

EXERCISE – DEVELOPING PARTIAL AND INSTRUMENTAL GOALS

Treatment as practiced by most helping service workers is psychosocial in nature. Treatment inventions for this global kind of work requires evaluation. In order to evaluate new procedures the social inventor must develop *partial goals*, steps to the more global final goal; and *instrumental goals*, assumed by worker and/or client to lead to the final goal by some indirect means.

Example – *Global psychosocial goal* =

– Commitment in relationship with opposite sex

Partial goal =

— revealing feelings to person of opposite sex
— finding out interests of dating partner
— making sacrifices of personal comfort for partner of opposite sex.

Example — *Global psychosocial goal* =

— Occupational competence

Instrumental goal =

— cooperation with work team members
— expressing opinions clearly and directly to boss and fellow workers
— listening empathically to fellow workers
— taking courses in listening skills and team membership.

Below are a number of global psychosocial goals. Using your imagination develop at least two partial and two instrumental goals for each.

Global psychosocial goal =

Increased self-esteem

Partial goal:

1. _____
   _____
2. _____
   _____

Instrumental goal:

1. _____
   _____
2. _____
   _____

Global psychosocial goal =

Ability to communicate on intimate level

Partial goal:
1. _____
   _____
2. _____
   _____

Instrumental goal:
1. _____
   _____
2. _____
   _____

Global psychosocial goal =
Capacity to trust friends
Partial goal:
1. _____
   _____
2. _____
   _____

Instrumental goal:
1. _____
   _____
2. _____
   _____

Global psychosocial goal =
Improve parental role
Partial goal:
1. _____
   _____
2. _____
   _____

Instrumental goal:
1. _____
   _____
2. _____
   _____

EXERCISE – EFFECTIVENESS, EFFICIENCY AND PROCESS

Inventive social programs seek validity and value for resources spent (dollars, time and manpower). In addition evaluation researchers want to know *how* they achieved these important goals. They want to scrutinize the program's process to be able to discover what parts and conditions of the program were most valuable in promoting program success.

In this exercise consider yourself an evaluation researcher who wants to view these criteria for evaluation. A brief description of a social program invention will be provided. Its control or comparison will also be described. Provide one indicator for measuring its effectiveness, efficiency and part of its process. Try to be as concrete in operationalizing the measure as you can.

> *Inventive Social Program* – group home for adolescents between ages 14-18, co-educational, use of mentor concept – each child is allowed to choose a staff member as his/her mentor; home consists of eight adolescents and six staff which includes the director who may be chosen as a mentor; mentors provide guidance, enforce rules of home and counseling; global goal of program is independent living by eighteenth birthday.

> *Comparison Social Program* – program is the same except for major difference that each child is *assigned* a staff member as their worker who is required to guide, enforce rules and counsel.

Effectiveness measure_____

_____

Efficiency measure_____

_____

Process measure_____

_____

Chapter 11

Inventing for the Helping Services

Knowledge for understanding socioeconomic, political and psychological phenomena frequently has been borrowed by the helping services from these respective fields (Kadushin, 1959). So too have methods for helping service practice. Psychoanalytic procedure, behavior modification techniques and family therapy methods have been borrowed and introduced into the body of helping service practices.

Recently, Thomas has suggested that the generation of social science findings, through the use of the behavioral science model, has not been effective in adding to the store of helping service technology (1978, p. 96). What the helping services requires, Thomas says, is a model of research that specifically relates to this professional need. Thomas calls his model, to be used for this purpose, Developmental Research and Utilization (DR&U). Rothman (1980), too, has proposed a model with similar purpose. Called Social Research and Development (Social R&D), the process is similar to an industrial R&D model in that it attempts to transform findings from the sciences into pragmatic applications for use in the everyday world.

These writers are occupied with the production of *social invention* for the helping services. What is social invention? Conger defines it *as the process whereby procedures, organizational arrangements and laws are freshly created to change the ways in which people relate to themselves or to each other* (1974, p. 1). Other labels for social invention are "social innovation" and "new social technology." "Social invention," however, is the term I will use to stand for the process that helps reach the helping service's professional end—that of providing better services to clientele through improved technical means.

What are some examples of social inventions? They are such things as the development of new social treatment techniques; new ways to assess client psychosocial status; various approaches to redesign agency organizational structure and the development of new social policy proposals, e.g., a national family social policy.

Consider the following as an example of a social invention:

> A worker *notices* that several clients have experienced the death of close family members and have been unable to grieve for them appropriately. Noting also that these clients are able to display sadness and grief upon the death of political figures and celebrities evidently meaningful to them, the helper constructs a socio-behavioral procedure whereby the clients can *transfer* their grief from these more distant figures to those more emotionally near.

In this social invention the helping service worker makes use of knowledge flexibly and creatively. By using knowledge of behavioral principles, primarily response shaping, and by using knowledge of the grief process the worker produces a new procedure for practice.

Within the last seven years I have taught a course in undergraduate social work that enables students to invent procedures, programs and policies for the helping service professions. A course assignment asks that social work students use the total CPS process for producing a prototype of a social invention. The following are a few of the inventions produced by these students:

1. an audio-visual demonstration of the effects of burnout, with an accompanying presentation of how various relaxation procedures can counteract job-related stress;
2. an environmental design kit for probation settings. The kit can be used by probationers to redesign the probation office milieu. It considers such factors as seating arrangements, office furniture and objects and colors and textures;
3. a new course for introduction into the social work curriculum.

This course emphasizes inter-disciplinary team work in the community change process, and

4. a treatment program for children who have been exposed to racial discrimination. The program is accompanied by guidelines so that it can be adopted by various social agencies.

A HELPING SERVICE METHOD FOR INVENTION

As mentioned above, Thomas has developed a model for inventing helping service technology. Table 4 shows the phases and operational steps of the DR&U process. In the table each operational step is accompanied by an example that has been taken from the making of an actual social invention.

The social invention process, as defined by Thomas, consists of five phases. Within each of these phases are a number of operational steps that must be completed. As can be seen in Table 4 there are a total of eleven operations necessary to complete the DR&U process.

Let's take a look at the DR&U process in action. The example used, that of the making of a training kit for welfare receptionists, did not, however, benefit from the use of the DR&U model. The kit, invented in 1972, did go through a process highly similar to that of DR&U. In developing the kit I was only partially aware of the kinds of steps necessary for invention. The kit was developed for a large governmental unit administering social services on a provincial level in Canada. In the example that follows I will take each operational *step* of the DR&U process and match it with the *actions* that I took in developing the kit.

1. Problem selection. The problem that was selected was: "How can we help welfare receptionists—First Contact Persons— become more sensitive to the needs of the clients they are receiving?" Welfare receptionists literally have first contact with the client. This first interaction then could significantly determine the client's perception of the welfare agency and the future course of the client's relationship with it.
2. Selection of information source. To learn more about the se-

lected problem I identified a number of probable sources of useful information. Selected to interview were welfare receptionists, various industries that had experience in training receptionists, the telephone company (because of their extensive experience in telephone communications), welfare administrators and clients.

3. Information gathering and evaluation. Interviews were had with all sources identified, with the exception of the clients. Written material was also obtained from the telephone company. Information from all sources was evaluated and four problematic themes were identified — (1) welfare receptionists did not understand the social welfare system as an institution and did not hold values similar to those of the helping services; (2) the receptionists became frustrated and angry when confronted with client anger; (3) the ethnic diversity of the welfare clientele made it difficult for receptionists to understand the client's behavior and values and (4) welfare receptionists required better communication skills, particularly those of empathy and concreteness, to promote a beginning relationship between client and agency.

4. & 5. Innovation of product: Product realization. Based upon this data, a First Contact Person prototype was constructed. It consisted of an interactive manual on the social welfare system which included information on welfare programs at all jurisdictional levels, their aims, and the means to reach them. The manual was designed to involve the reader and included questions, games and self-testing procedures. The kit also included audio exercises in empathy and concreteness in which users received immediate taped feedback on their performance. Audio exercises were also developed for dealing with the problem of client anger. The kit's final component was an exercise aimed to induce stereotypical reactions to clients by looking at photographs of ethnic scenes and persons. The exercise attempted to help receptionists look underneath the surface of presenting characteristics of persons and their environments to perceive individual uniqueness and also the commonality between all persons. The kit was self-administering and designed to be completed in five two-hour sessions.

6. Trial use. At completion the kit was administered to five welfare receptionists in five different geographical regions.
7. & 8. Collection of evaluative data. Evaluation of product. Research scales were constructed to receive welfare receptionists' reactions to the various components of the kit. As well, detailed interviews were held with the receptionists. Information received from these interviews proved to be valuable in making changes in the kit's construction.
9. Preparation of diffusion media. Following the redesign of the kit, a brochure was prepared to describe the purposes and features of the kit.
10. Dissemination of production information. Brochures were mailed to all welfare administrators in each district office within the jurisdiction.
11. Implementation by users. First Contact Person Kits were mailed upon request to over sixty offices for use by welfare receptionists. (Evaluation of welfare receptionists' reactions to the kit was made by including within the kit package a self-administering questionnaire that attempted to tap the kit's training effectiveness. A report was compiled from the returning data. The evaluation of the kit was found to be moderately to highly favorable. Operations 7 and 8 repeated.)

As can be seen my actions as a social inventor came relatively close to the steps that Thomas has identified as components of the DR&U process.

Let's look closely at the DR&U model. What most of the model most nearly resembles is a problem-solving model. Similarity exists between DR&U's first three phases and most normative problem-solving models. The DR&U model differs from problem-solving models by including diffusion and adoption phases. The product must be marketed and, in a word, consumed.

Gaps in the DR&U Model

Thomas's DR&U model offers valuable guidelines for the development of new social technology. It identifies the various *phases* and *operations* that the social inventor can follow toward the goal of

TABLE 4. Phases and operations of the DR&U model with examples of the models' operations. Used with permission of University of Chicago Press. Edwin Thomas, "Mousetraps, Developmental Research, and Social Work Education." *Social Service Review*, Vol. 52, No. 3, Sept., 1978.

PHASE	OPERATION	EXAMPLE
ANALYSIS	1. Problem selection	→ How to make welfare receptionists more sensitive to clients?
	2. Selection of information source	→ Welfare administrators; Bell Telephone; Business and Industries.
DEVELOPMENT	3. Information gathering and evaluation	→ Welfare administrators interviewed; information from Bell Telephone and industries read.
	4. Innovation of product	→ Components of product identified --anger; communication skills; ethnicity; welfare information.
	5. Product realization	→ Audio visual kit with accompanying book on social welfare.
EVALUATION	6. Trial use	→ Welfare receptionists selected for kit administration; kit administered.
	7. Collection of evaluative data	→ Research scales filled out by welfare receptionists; interviews conducted.
	8. Evaluation of product	→ Data evaluated and changes made in product due to data feedback.
DIFFUSION	9. Preparation of diffusion media	→ Brochure written describing features and purpose of kit.
	10. Dissemination of product information	→ Brochures mailed to potential users.
ADOPTION	11. Implementation by users	→ Requests filled and mailed to users; welfare receptionists trained with kit.

realizing new social technology. Further, the model indicates that the social inventor or invention team requires a host of skills, e.g., information retrieval, creative application of data, design abilities, research capabilities and marketing aptitude, if the goal of utilization of new social technology is to be reached. These points are strong merits in the model's favor.

My major concern with the model is this — that it treats the development of social technology without consideration of the creative *attitudes* and *aptitudes* that are necessary for its realization. Thomas does recognize that what he calls *the generation process*, i.e., the transformation, adaptation, conversion, extension, or specific application of information sources for invention, calls for an understanding of how these activities are done. He states:

> The critical activities involved in the generating process require future analysis, explication, and conceptualization because they are undoubtedly among the distinctive research methods of developmental research. Because the essential activities involved in treating and assembling information from the basic sources and in generating social technology from the information are at the heart of developmental research, they themselves should be the subject of methodological and analysis and inquiry. (1978, p. 113)

But it is not only in the generation process that the DR&U model fails to adopt a creative stance. Consider the first operational step within the model, *problem selection*. How does the developmental researcher or research team select the problem to be solved? Thomas tells us that:

> at the outset, before any developmental activity occurs, there is some problematic human condition involving potential social welfare clientele for which one possible direction for change is the development of social technology. (1978, p. 106)

Problematic human conditions arise out of *need*. A problem is selected because it is viewed as arising from a condition of human need. Problem selection must, however, be rooted in the idea that need can be used as a jumping-off place to define a myriad of problems based upon this basic need. What is required in problem selection is the *divergent search* that leads to many problem definitions based upon this identification of one need. The problem-finding methods and activities identified and discussed and elaborated in Chapter 5 are necessary for a creative approach to problem selection. Divergent methodology is useful in finding problems that are not merely obvious.

Therefore, my view of the DR&U model is this—it is a rational, sequential problem-solving model that excludes the thinking activities, divergent and convergent, that are required for a creative approach to social invention. DR&U is essentially a model in search of a *creative* method.

ROTHMAN'S SOCIAL R&D MODEL

Jack Rothman (1980) has conceived a model for social invention, which he calls the Social Research and Development Model (Social R&D). Rothman has produced a clearly explicated model that differs from Thomas's in that Rothman perceives the process of social innovation as strictly tied to the conversion of *social science findings* to prescriptive guidelines for helping service practice. Rothman's model (see Figure 49) counts upon search and retrieval methodology. He works by seeking consensus generalizations that can be drawn from a body of research. One such generalization is found in Rothman's attempts to tease out the practice prescription that may be suggested within it. For example, social science findings converge upon this generalization—that the less talking one does in a small group situation the less power one is perceived as having within it (Bednar, Weet, Evensen, Lanier & Melnick,

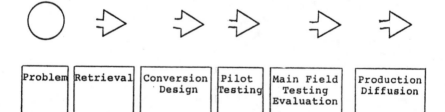

FIGURE 49. The social R&D method.

1974). Therefore, a prescription would suggest that group leaders, to encourage an equivalent distribution of power within a group, must encourage non-talkers to meaningfully participate. Individual sessions might be set up between the talker and quiet, withdrawn members to support such new behavior.

Rothman has made an important contribution to both helping service practice and the social invention process by focusing upon the utilization of knowledge already accumulated within social science domains. His model serves a necessary function: the integration of useful empirical data into the social work knowledge base for practice.

There are difficulties in using his model. Rothman has noted problems that social work and social science students have in transforming consensus generalizations into prescriptive guidelines for practice (1980, p. 102). I believe these problems arise from student inability to *play* with the data and may also be specifically related to a lack of fluency and flexibility in divergent thinking. Rothman briefly has mentioned the possible use of creative methods to improve the social inventor's ability in this area (1980, pp. 103-104.)

Patti, in his rigorous review of Rothman's model, has identified what appears to be a serious flaw in the Social R&D Model. Because the model concerns itself *only* with the search for social science data that relate to the problem at hand, Patti argues that:

> a religious adherence to the model might tempt the R&D specialist to choose only those problems for which there is a social science research. This would be a clear case of means determining ends. A more flexible and ultimately more useful way to proceed in this early stage would be to draw upon whatever sources of information appear relevant to the goal or problem at hand. (1981, p. 40)

I agree with Patti. Focusing only upon social science data can be severely limiting to the social invention process. Ideas for social invention can be gained by surveying a range of knowledge and practice domains, both inside and outside the social science boundaries. That many social inventions have been conceived by individuals only marginally affiliated with the helping services and also relatively ignorant of the social science literature suggests that social inventions can be triggered by many different stimuli. The invention of Alcoholics Anonymous, various other self-help addiction programs, e.g., diet, gambling, smoking, etc., and the Boy Scouts, are examples of social inventions coming from individuals outside of the professional helping service framework (Conger, 1974). The social settlement house movement, a social invention that led to many other creative social innovations, e.g., child labor laws, vocational guidance, group work, etc., was developed without the benefit of a sound social science data base, indicating that strong purpose and the ability to *notice* social phenomena, along with the capacity to generate good ideas in response to these social needs can be effective instruments for making social innovation (Davis, 1967).

Rothman's Social R&D Model is strong on retrieval of data from the social sciences. He has elaborated a methodology for retrieving data from social science research. His model, however, must be considered of limited usefulness to the social inventor because of the boundaries it places around knowledge for social invention. Further the model's lack of employment of creative methods, as defined in this book, may prevent it from having greater impact than so far illustrated.

SOCIAL INVENTIONS—DIFFICULT TO PRODUCE

Social invention is relatively infrequent in the helping services. Why? What are some of the obstacles that stand in the way of developing new approaches to helping service practice? Here, I am not talking about the obstacles that stand in the way of creativity—psychological, socioeconomic and characterological—rather these are blocks that have been generated by the way in which helping service agencies and educational institutions operate. They are obstacles produced, in some cases, because of the present sociopolitical milieu. Let's consider some of these obstacles in brief.

1. *Efficiency vs. Process*—Watson (1983) has noted that an overemphasis upon efficient administrative practices within the helping agencies has led to a relative de-emphasis upon process-oriented activities. This focus upon practice that is efficient and accountable unfortunately has promoted attitudes

that are very much against "reinventing the wheel." Agencies with a strong efficiency orientation take over from the business sector tend to play it safe, becoming wedded to the preservation of the status quo.

2. *Helping Service Curricula* —Helping service curricula, although they address the notion of social innovation, in the main, do not include the methodology of social invention nor the knowledge and methods developed in the field of creative education.

3. *Social Science Knowledge* —Knowledge generated in the social sciences is often difficult to transform into useable form. Some of this knowledge, although potentially of value, must be carefully culled (à la Rothman) for generalizations that can be turned into utilizable guidelines for practice. The difficulty, in part, is related to the kind of findings generated in social science. Because the social sciences are young disciplines that use imprecise (frequently unreliable and invalid) measuring devices, the findings that are identified are ofttimes conflicting, leading to the inability to form consensus generalizations. Further, research designs involving people are very difficult to replicate. Differences in study design can lead to variable study results, again creating a situation where conflicting research results in a study area make generalizing about it untenable.

What further confounds this difficulty inherent in the existing social science knowledge base is the lack of skill that helping service students have in *transforming* consensus generalizations into practice prescription. This problem can be resolved by introducing knowledge and method from creative education into the social work curriculum. Evidence suggests that creativity tends to fall off after undergraduate education (Simonton, 1983). Creative education in social work may reverse any tendency for advanced education to make students less fluent and flexible thinkers.

4. *Absence of a Social Invention Stance* —Social scientists and social work academicians infrequently take a stance favoring social invention. In the main they perceive their role to be that of knowledge builder. They generally assume a disinterested

pose toward the knowledge they generate. It has been esti-
mated that the first major impact of a social science break-
through takes between 10 to 15 years after it has been achieved
(Deutch et al., 1971). If social science and helping service
academicians were to take a greater interest in the diffusion
and adoption of social inventions this time lag might be decreased.

5. *Public Apathy Toward Social Technology* — High technology
clearly has the attention of the general public today. The emphasis upon sensational breakthroughs in computer and electronic technology has commanded a broad interest. Clearly
there is less interest in the development of social technology,
even though it may be true that high tech advances may require
social technology to ameliorate their unintended consequences. For example, it appears that computer technology
and robotics will make many jobs superfluous in the near future. How can we solve the problem of distributing income
equitably in a society that will require a smaller work force?
Or a work force in which there will be a need for a relatively
small but highly trained technical group and a large group of
minimally trained service workers. The general public's and
government's lack of interest in such powerful social issues
prevents many inventive social scientists from involving themselves in issues for which research funding is highly unlikely
to be found.

6. *A Changing Public Mood* — Going hand in hand with the public's lack of interest in the development of social technology is
the public's view that social problems such as poverty, unemployment, family breakdown and crime are predominantly the
fault of the individual. Whereas the view of the public during
the turbulent 60s was toward an environmental explanation of
social dysfunction, today the pendulum has swung toward the
pole of individual causation. Social history is replete with examples of the cyclical nature of social reform and social con-
servatism. The public perceives social problems today as
rooted in failings of individual character. Such a change in the
public's perception of social phenomena can only hinder interest and motivation in the nurturing of social invention.

The factors noted above are some of the most potent ones blocking the development of new social technology. As can be seen some of the factors are *internal* to helping service professions, whereas others, such as government and public disinterest, are clearly *external* to it. Clearly there is an interactive effect between these factors. Public and governmental indifference to social innovation does not provide the support, both financial and moral, to carry forward with an inventive spirit. The interactive mix of internal and external blocks to social invention is potent. Nevertheless, there is some cause for optimism. Tools for social invention such as CPS, DR&U and Social R&D when coupled with a group of highly purposeful and creative helping service educators, practitioners and students can keep alive the spirit of social invention.

Summary

Social inventions are the development of new procedures, organizational arrangements and laws. CPS provides both model and method for their development. Thomas's DR&U model and Rothman's model of Social R&D provide alternative maps for reaching the objective of social invention. I have contended that only an integration of *model* with *creative method* can *best* reach the social invention goal. This chapter has also provided a brief discussion of some of the factors involved in impeding the social invention process in the social sciences and the helping services.

ADDITIONAL READINGS

A. D. Moore. *Invention, Discovery and Creativity*, New York: Doubleday, 1969.

Robert D. Boyd and Allen Menlo. "Solving Problems of Practice in Education: A Prescriptive Model For the Use of Scientific Information." *Knowledge*, Vol. 6, No. 1, September, 1984, pp. 59-73.

Ronald G. Havelock, *Planning for Innovation through Dissemination and Utilization of Knowledge*. Ann Arbor: Institute for Social Research, University of Michigan, 1973.

Bibliography

Ackerman, N., Beatman, F., and Sherman, S. *Exploring the Base for Family Therapy*. New York: Family Service Association of America, 1961.

Adams, James L. *Conceptual Blockbusting: A Guide to Better Ideas*. San Francisco: W. H. Freeman, 1974.

Alamshah, William H. "Blockages to Creativity." *Journal of Creative Behavior*, Vol. 6, No. 2, 1972, pp. 105-113.

Anderson, Barry F. *The Complete Thinker*. Englewood Cliffs, New Jersey: Prentice-Hall, 1980.

Arieti, Silvano. *Interpretation of Schizophrenia*. New York: Brunner, 1955.

Arieti, Silvano. *Creativity – The Magic Synthesis*. New York: Basic Books, 1976.

Barron, Frank. "The Disposition Toward Originality." *The Journal of Abnormal and Social Psychology*, Vol. 51, No. 3, 1955, pp. 478-485.

Barron, Frank. *Creativity and Personal Freedom*. Princeton, N. J.: Van Nostrand, 1968.

Basadur, Min, Graen, George B., and Green, Stephen G. "Training in Creative Problem Solving: Effects on Ideation and Problem Finding and Solving in an Industrial Research Organization." *Organizational Behavior and Human Performance*, Vol. 30, 1982, pp. 41-70.

Bateson, G., Jackson, D., Haley, J., and Weakland, J. "Toward a Theory of Schizophrenia." *Behavioral Science*, Vol. 1, No. 4, 1956, pp. 251-264.

Bednar, Richard L., Weet, Connie, Evensen, Paul, Lanier, David, Melnick, Joseph. "Empirical Guidelines for Group Therapy: Pretraining, Cohesion, and Modeling." *Journal of Applied Behavioral Science*, Vol. 10, No. 2, 1974, pp. 149-165.

Bennett, Carl A. and Lumsdaine, Arthur A. (Eds). *Evaluation and Experiment: Some Critical Issues in Assessing Social Programs*. New York: Academic Press, 1975.

Berman, Jeffrey S. and Norton, Nicholas C. "Does Professional Training Make a Therapist More Effective?" *Psychological Bulletin*, Vol. 98, No. 2, 1985, pp. 401-407.

Biestek, Felix P. *The Casework Relationship*. Chicago: Loyola University Press, 1957.

Birney, Robert. *Fear of Failure*. New York: Van Nostrand-Reinhold, 1969.

Bloom, Martin. *The Paradox of Helping: Introduction to the Philosophy of Scientific Practice*. New York: John Wiley and Sons, 1975.

Boyd, Robert D. and Menlo, Allen. "Solving Problems of Practice in Education: A Prescriptive Model For the Use of Scientific Information." *Knowledge*, Vol. 6, No. 1, September, 1984, pp. 59-73.

Brager, George and Holloway, Stephen. *Changing Human Service Organizations: Politics and Practice*. New York: The Free Press, 1978.

Brickner, William H. and Cope, Donald M. *The Planning Process*. Cambridge, Mass.: Winthrop, 1977.

Brown, R. V., Rahr, A. S., and Peterson, C. *Decision-Analysis for the Manager*. New York: Holt, Rinehart and Winston, 1974.

Brunner, Jerome S. *Beyond the Information Given*. New York: Norton, 1973.

Campbell, Donald T. and Stanley, Julian C. *Experimental and Quasi-Experimental Designs for Research*. Chicago: Rand McNally, 1963.

Caro, Francis G. (Ed.). *Readings in Evaluation Research*, 2nd Ed., New York: Russell Sage, 1977.

Cole, H. P., and Lacefield, W. E. "Skill Domains Critical to the Helping Professions." *Personnel and Guidance Journal*, Vol. 57, 1978, pp. 115-123.

Compton, Beulah R. and Galaway, Burt. *Social Work Processes*, 3rd edition. Chicago: The Dorsey Press, 1984.

Conger D. Stuart. *Social Inventions*. Saskatoon: Modern Press, 1974.

Crutchfield, R. S. "Nurturing the Cognitive Skills of Productive Thinking." In *Life Skills in School and Society*. Washington, D.C.: Association for Supervision and Curriculum Development, 1969.

Csikszentmihalyi, M. and Getzels, J. W. "Discovery-Oriented Behavior and the Originality of Creative Products: A Study with Artists." *Journal of Personality and Social Psychology*, Vol. 19, No. 1, 1971, pp. 47-52.

Davis, Allen F. *Spearheads for Reform: The Social Settlements and the Progressive Movement 1890-1914*. New York: Oxford University Press, 1967.

de Bono, Edward. *Lateral thinking: A Textbook of Creativity*. Middlesex, England: Penguin Books, 1977.

Delbecq, Andre L., Van de Ven, Andrew H., Gustafson, David H. *Group Techniques for Program Planning: A Guide to Nominal Group and Delphi Processes*. Glenview, Ill.: Scott, Foresman and Col., 1975.

Dellas, M. and Gaier, E. L. "Identification of Creativity: The Individual." *Psychological Bulletin*, Vol. 73, No. 1, 1970, pp. 55-73.

Deutsch, Karl. W., Platt, John, and Senghaas. "Conditions Favoring Major Advances in Science." *Science*, Vol. 3, 1971, pp. 450-459.

Dewey, John. *How We Think*, rev. ed. New York: D.C. Heath, 1933.

Dillon, J. T. "The Multidisciplinary Study of Questioning." *Journal of Educational Psychology*, Vol. 74, 1982, pp. 147-165.

Dillon, J. T. "Problem Finding and Solving." *Journal of Creative Behavior*, Vol. 16, No. 2, 1982, pp. 97-111.

Dixon, David, Heppner, P. Paul, Petersen, Chris H., and Ronning, Royce R. "Problem-Solving Workshop Training." *Journal of Counseling Psychology*, Vol. 26, No. 2, 1979, pp. 133-139.

Dror, Yehezkel. "The Planning Process: A Facet Design." In *Planning-Programming-Budgeting* (Eds.), Fremond J. Lyden and Ernest G. Miller. Chicago: Markham Publishing Co., 1967, pp. 93-116.

D'Zurilla, Thomas J. and Goldfried, Marvin, R. "Problem Solving and Behavior Modification." *Journal of Abnormal Psychology*, Vol 78, No. 1, 1971, pp. 107-126.

D'Zurilla, Thomas J. and Nezu, Arthur. "A Study of the Generation-of-Alternatives Processes in Social Problem Solving." *Cognitive Therapy and Research*, Vol. 4, No. 1, 1980, pp. 67-72.

Einstein, A. and Infeld, L. *The Evolution of Physics*. New York: Simon and Schuster, 1938.

Epstein, Irwin, and Tripodi, Tony. *Research Techniques for Program Planning, Monitoring and Evaluation*. New York: Columbia University Press, 1977.

Eysenck, Hans J. "The Roots of Creativity: Cognitive Ability or Personality Trait?" *Roeper Review*, Vol. 5, No. 4, April-May, 1983.

Fairweather, George W. *Methods for Experimental Social Innovation*. New York: John Wiley and Sons, 1967.

Falck, Hans. "A Loud and Shrill Protest." *Journal of Education for Social Work*, Vol. 20, No. 2, Sept., 1984, pp. 3-4.

Fortune, Anne E. "Problem-Solving Ability of Social Work Students." *Journal of Education for Social Work*, Vol. 20, No. 2, 1984, pp. 25-33.

Freud, Sigmund. "The Relation of the Poet to Day-Dreaming." Collected Papers, 4, New York: Basic Books, 1959a, pp. 173-183.

Freud, Sigmund. "Formulation Regarding the Two Principles in Mental Functioning." Collected Papers, 4, New York: Basic Books, 1959b, pp. 13-21.

Gelfand, Bernard. "Creative Imagination: The Forgotten Ingredient in Social Work Practice." *Journal of Education for Social Casework*, Vol. 63, No. 8, Oct., 1982a, pp. 499-503.

Gelfand, Bernard. "Nurturing Integrated Brain Hemispheric Functioning in Undergraduate Social Work Students." *Journal of Education for Social Work*, Vol. 18, No. 1, Winter, 1982b, pp. 43-50.

Gelfand, Bernard. "Toward an Integration of Creative Problem Solving Methodology with the Developmental Research and Utilization Model." *Canadian Journal of Social Work Education*, Vol. 8, No. 3, 1982c, pp. 47-57.

Getzels, J. W. "Problem-Finding and the Inventiveness of Solutions." *Journal of Creative Behavior*, Vol. 9, No. 1, 1975, pp. 12-18.

Getzels, J. W. "The Problem of the Problem." In *Question Framing and Response Consistency* (Ed.), P. M. Hogarth. San Francisco: Jossey-Bass, 1982.

Ghiselin, Brewster. "Ultimate Criteria for Two Levels of Creativity." In *Scientific Creativity: Its Recognition and Development* (Eds.), Calvin W. Taylor and Frank Barron, New York: John Wiley and Sons, 1964.

Gilbert, Neil and Specht, Harry. *Planning for Social Welfare.* Englewood Cliffs, N.J.: Prentice-Hall, 1977.

Goffman, Erving. *Asylums: Essays on the Social Situation of Mental Patients and Other Inmates*. Garden City, N.Y.: Doubleday, 1961.

Googins, B., Capoccia, V. A., and Kaufman, N. "The Interactional Dimension of Planning: A Framework for Practice." *Social Work*, Vol. 28, No. 4, July-August, 1983, pp. 273-277.

Gordon, Rosemary. "A Very Private World." In *The Function and Nature of Imagery* (Ed.), Peter W. Sheehan, New York: Academic Press, 1972.

Gordon, William J. J. *Synectics: The Development of Creative Capacity*. New York: Collier Books, 1961.

Guilford, J. P. *The Nature of Human Intelligence*. New York: Mc-Graw-Hill, 1967.

Guilford, J. P., Hendricks, Moana, and Hoepfner, Ralph. "Solving Social Problems Creatively." *Journal of Creative Behavior*, Vol. 2, No. 3, 1968, pp. 155-164.

Guilford, J. P. *Way Beyond the I.Q.* Buffalo, New York: Creative Education Foundation, 1977.

Guilford, J. P. "Some Incubated Thoughts on Incubation." *Journal of Creative Behavior*, Vol. 13, No. 1, 1979, pp. 1-8.

Haley, Jay. *Problem-Solving Therapy: New Strategies for Effective Family Therapy*. San Francisco: Jossey-Bass, 1976.

Hallowitz, David. "The Problem-Solving Component in Family Therapy." *Social Casework*, Vol. 51, No. 2, Feb., 1970, pp. 67-75.

Havelock, Ronald G. *Planning for Innovation Through Dissemina-*

Heppner, P. Paul. "A Review of the Problem-Solving Literature and its Relationship to the Counseling Process." *Journal of Counseling Psychology*, Vol. 25, No. 5, 1978, pp. 366-375.

Hepworth, Dean H. and Larsen, Jo Ann. 2nd edition. *Direct Social Work Practice: Theory and Skills*. Chicago: The Dorsey Press, 1986.

Hersen, M. and Barlow, D. H. *Single-Case Experimental Designs: Strategies For Studying Behavior Change*. New York: Pergamon Press, 1976.

Howard, Darlene V. *Cognitive Psychology: Memory, Language and Thought*. New York: MacMillan Publishing Co., 1983, Chapter 12, Problem Solving.

Hudson, L. *Contrary Imaginations*. London: Penguin, 1966.

Jayaratne, Srinika and Levy, Rona L. *Empirical Clinical Practice*. New York: Columbia University Press, 1979.

Johnson, Louise C. *Social Work Practice: A Generalist Approach*. Boston: Allyn and Bacon, 1983.

Kadushin, Alfred. "The Knowledge of Social Work." In *Issues in American Social Work* (Ed.), Alfred J. Kahn. New York: Columbia University Press, 1959, pp. 39-79.

Kadushin, Alfred. "Diagnosis and Evaluation for (Almost) All Occasions." *Social Work*, Vol. 8, No. 1, 1963, pp. 12-19.

Kagle, Jill Doner. "Evaluating Social Work Practice." *Social Work*, Vol. 24, No. 4, July, 1979, pp. 292-296.

Kepner C. H. and Tregoe, B. B. *The Rational Manager: A Systematic Approach to Problem Solving and Decision-Making*. New York: McGraw-Hill, 1965.

Khatena, Joe. "Identification and Stimulation of Creative Imagination Imagery." *Journal of Creative Behavior*, Vol. 12, No. 1, 1978, pp. 30-38.

Khatena, Joe. *Imagery and Creative Imagination*. Buffalo, New York: Bearly Ltd., 1984.

Klau, Eleanor. "The Effect of a Three-Day Workshop in Creative Problem on Selected Aspects of Problem-Solving Ability in Graduate Students of Social Work. Unpublished doctoral dissertation, University of Maryland, 1981.

Klau, Eleanor and Gelfand, Bernard. "Changes in Students' Creative Problem-solving Abilities and Their Implications for Social Work Eduction." Unpublished manuscript, 1984.

Kochler, C. T. "Project Planning and Management Technique." *Public Administration Review*, Vol. 43, No. 5, September-October, 1983, pp. 459-466.

Kolb, David A., Rubin, Irwin M., and McIntyre, James M. *Organizational Psychology: An Experiential Approach*, 2nd ed., Englewood Cliffs, N.J.: Prentice-Hall, 1974.

Kris, Ernst. *Psychoanalytic Explorations in Art*. London: Allen and Irwin, 1954.

Lippitt, Gordon L. *Visualizing Change: Model Building and the Change Process*. La Jolla, California: University Associates, 1973.

Maeroff, Gene. "Teaching to Think: A New Emphasis." *The New York Times Winter Survey in Education*. January 9, 1983.

MacKinnon, Donald W. "The Nature and Nurture of Creative Talent." *American Psychologist*, Vol. 17, 1962, pp. 484-495.

MacKinnon, Donald W. "Personality Correlates of Creativity." In *Productive Thinking in Education* (Eds.), M. J. Aschner and C. E. Bish. Washington, D.C.: *National Education Association*, 1965, pp. 158-171.

MacKinnon, Donald W. *In Search of Human Effectiveness: Identifying and Developing Creativity*. Buffalo, N.Y.: Creative Education Foundation, 1978.

Mahoney, Michael J. *Self-Change: Strategies for Solving Personal Problems*. New York: W. W. Norton, 1979.

March, James G. "Footnotes to Organizational Change." *Administrative Science Quarterly*, Vol. 26, No. 4, December, 1981, pp. 563-577.

Marsenich, Robert. "How to Teach the Steps of Change." *Training*, Vol. 20, No. 3, March, 1983, pp. 62-63.

Maslow, Abraham. "Emotional Blocks to Creativity." In *A Source Book for Creative Thinking* (Eds.), Sidney J. Parnes and Harold Harding. New York: Charles Scribner's Sons, 1962, pp. 94-103.

Maslow, Abraham. *Motivation and Personality*, 2nd ed., New York: Harper and Row, 1970.

Maslow, Abraham. *The Further Reaches of Human Nature*. New York: Viking Press, 1971.

McKim, Robert. "Relaxed Attention." In *Guide to Creative Action* (Eds.), Sidney J. Parnes, Ruth Noller and Angelo Biondi. New York: Charles Scribner's Sons, 1977, pp. 206-211.

McMullan, W. E. "Creative Individuals: Paradoxical Personages." *Journal of Creative Behavior*, Vol. 10, No. 4, 1976, pp. 265-275.

Meichenbaum, Donald. "Enhancing Creativity by Modifying What Subjects Say to Themselves." *American Educational Research Journal*, Vol. 12, No. 2, 1975, pp. 129-145.

Meyer, Henry J., Borgatta, Edgar F., and Jones, Wyatt C. *Girls at Vocational High*. New York: Russell Sage Foundation, 1965.

Minuchin, Salvador, Montalvo, B., Guerney, B. G., Jr., Rosman, B. L., and Schumer, F. (Eds.), *Families of the Slums*. New York: Basic Books, 1967.

Moore, A. D. *Invention Discovery and Creativity*. New York: Doubleday, 1969.

Nelsen, Judith C. "Issues in Single-Subject Research for Non-Behaviorists." *Social Work Research and Abstracts*, Vol. 17, No. 1, Spring, 1981, pp. 31-37.

Nezu, Arthur and D'Zurilla, Thomas J. "An Experimental Evaluation of the Decision-Making Process in Solving Problem Solving." *Cognitive Therapy and Research*, Vol. 3, 1979, pp. 269-277.

Nezu, Arthur and D'Zurilla, Thomas J. "Effects of Problem Definition and Formulation on Decision Making in the Social Problem-Solving Process." *Behavior Therapy*, Vol. 12, No. 1, 1981a, pp. 100-106.

Nezu, Arthur and D'Zurilla, Thomas J. H. "Effects of Problem Definition and Formulation on the Generation of Alternatives in the Social Problem-Solving Process." *Cognitive Therapy and Research*, Vol. 5, No. 3, 1981b, pp. 265-271.

Northen, Helen. *Clinical Social Work*. New York: Columbia University Press, 1981.

Osborn, Alex. *Applied Imagination*, 3rd ed. New York: Charles Scribner's Sons, 1963.

Noller, Ruth, Parnes, Sidney J., and Biondi, Angelo M. *Creative Actions Book*. New York: Charles Scribner's Sons, 1976.

Papanek, Victor, J. "Tree of Life: Bionics." *Journal of Creative Behavior*, Vol. 3, No. 1, 1969, pp. 5-15.

Papanek, Victor. *Design for the Real World*. Toronto: Bantam Books, 1973.

Parnes, Sidney J. and Meadows, Arnold. "Effects of 'Brainstorming' Instructions on Creative Problem-Solving by Trained and Untrained Subjects." *Journal of Educational Psychology*, Vol. 50, No. 4, 1958, pp. 171-176.

Parnes, Sidney J. "Toward a Better Understanding of Brainstorming." In *The Creative Process* (Ed.), Angelo M. Biondi, Buffalo, N.Y.: *D.O.K.*, pp. 33-45.

Parnes, Sidney J. and Biondi, Angelo M. "Creative Behavior: A Delicate Balance." *Journal of Creative Behavior*, Vol. 9, No. 3, 1975, pp. 149-157.

Parnes, Sidney J. "CPSI: The General System." *Journal of Creative Behavior*, Vol. 11, No. 1, 1977, pp. 1-11.

Parnes, Sidney J. *The Magic of Your Mind*. Buffalo, N.Y.: Creative Education Foundation, 1981.

Patti, Rino J. "The Prospects for Social R&D: An Essay Review." *Social Work Research and Abstracts*, Vol. 17, No. 2, Summer, 1981, pp. 38-44.

Perlman, Helen Harris. *Social Casework: A Problem Solving Process*. Chicago: The University of Chicago Press, 1957.

Perlman, Helen Harris. "The Problem-Solving Model in Social Casework." In *Theories of Social Casework* (Eds.), Robert W. Roberts and Robert H. Nee. Chicago: The University of Chicago Press, 1970, pp. 129-179.

Pincus, Allan and Minahan, Anne. *Social Work Practice: Model and Method*. Itasca, Ill.: F. E. Peacock, 1973.

Prince, George. *The Practice of Creativity*. New York: Collier Books, 1970.

Reid, William J. and Epstein, Laura. *Task-Centered Practice*. New York: Columbia University Press, 1972.

Reid, William J. and Epstein, Laura. *Task-Centered Practice*. New York: Columbia University Press, 1977.

Reid, William J. *The Task-Centered System*. New York: Columbia University Press, 1978.

232   THE CREATIVE PRACTITIONER

Reik, Theodor. *Listening With the Third Ear*. New York: Farrar, Straus and Company, 1949.

Reynolds. Bertha C. *Learning and Teaching in the Practice of Social Work*. New York: Farrar and Rinehart, Inc., 1942.

Rivlin, Alice. *Systematic Thinking for Social Action*. Washington, D.C.: Brookings, 1971.

Roe, Anne. "A Psychological Study of Eminent Biologists." *Psychological Monographs*, Vol. 65, No. 14, 1951, pp. 1-28.

Rogers, Carl. "The Necessary and Sufficient Conditions of Therapeutic Personality Change." *Journal of Consulting Psychology*. Vol. 21, 1957, pp. 95-103.

Rogers, Carl. "Toward a Theory of Creativity." In *A Source Book for Creative Thinking* (Eds.), Sidney J. Parnes and Harold Harding. New York: Charles Scribner's Sons, 1962, pp. 64-72.

Rothenberg, Albert. *The Emerging Goddess: The Creative Process in Art, Science and Other Fields*. Chicago: University of Chicago Press, 1979.

Rothman, Jack. *Social R&D: Research and Development in the Human Services*. Englewood Cliffs, N.J.: Prentice-Hall, Inc., 1980.

Rutman, Leonard (Ed). *Evaluation Research Methods*. Beverly Hills, Calif.: Sage Publications, 1977.

Satir, Virginia. *Conjoint Family Therapy*. Rev. ed. Palo Alto, Calif: Science and Behavior Books, 1967.

Schein, Edgar. *Professional Education*. New York: McGraw-Hill, 1973.

Schön, Donald. *The Reflective Practitioner: How Professionals Think in Action*. New York: Basic Books, 1983.

Schulman, Lawrence. *The Skills of Helping: Individuals and Groups*. Itasca, Ill.: F. E. Peacock, 1979.

Schwartz, Arthur and Goldiamond, Israel. *Social Casework: A Behavioral Approach*. New York: Columbia University Press, 1975.

Siegleman, Ellen Y. *Personal Risk: Mastering Change in Love and Work*. New York: Harper and Row, 1983.

Silveira, J. Incubation: The Effect of Interruption, *Timing and Length on Problem Solution and Quality of Problem Processing*. Unpublished doctoral dissertation, University of Oregon, 1971.

Simonton, Dean Keith. "Formal Education, Eminence and Dogmatism." *Journal of Creative Behavior*, Vol. 17, No. 3, 1983, pp. 149-162.

Smilansky, J. "Problem Solving and the Quality of Invention: An Empirical Investigation." *Journal of Educational Psychology*, Vol. 76, No. 3, pp. 377-386.

Sommer, Robert. *The Mind's Eye: Imagery in Everyday Life*. New York: Delta, 1968.

Spedale, Daniel R. "Reducing Resistance to Innovation." In *The Creative Process* (Ed.). Angelo M. Biondi. Buffalo, N.Y.: Creative Education Foundation, 1972, pp. 62-67.

Spitzer, Kurt and Walsh, Betty. "A Problem Focused Model of Practice." *Social Casework*, Vol. 50, No. 6, June, 1969, pp. 323-329.

Spivack, George and Platt, Jerome J. "Problem Solving Therapy: The Description of a New Program for Chronic Psychiatric Patients." *Psychotherapy; Theory, Research and Practice*, Vol. 13, No. 4, Winter, 1976, pp. 368-373.

Stein, Morris I. *Stimulating Creativity*, Vol. I. New York: Academic Press, 1974.

Stein, Morris I. *Stimulating Creativity*, Vol. II. New York: Academic Press, 1975.

Strean, Herbert S. *Clinical Social Work: Theory and Practice*. New York: The Free Press, 1978.

Suchman, Edward. *Evaluative Research*. New York: Russell Sage Foundation, 1967.

Taylor, Irving A. "An Emerging View of Creative Actions." In *Perspectives in Creativity* (Eds.), Irving A. Taylor and J. W. Getzels. Chicago: Aldine Publishing Co., 1975, pp. 297-325.

Thomas, Edwin J. "Generating Innovation in Social Work: The Paradigm of Developmental Research." *Journal of Social Service Research*, Vol. 2, No. 1, Fall, 1978, pp. 95-115.

Toseland, Ronald W., Rivas, Robert F., and Chapman, Dennis. "An Evaluation of Decision-Making in Task Groups." *Social Work*, Vol 29, No. 4, July-August, 1984, pp. 339-346.

Tripodi, Tony and Epstein, Irwin. *Research Techniques for Clinical Social Workers*. New York: Columbia University Press, 1980.

Truax, Charles B. and Carkhuff, Robert R. *Toward Effective Counseling and Psychotherapy: Training and Practice*. Chicago: Aldine, 1967.

Tumin, Melvin. "Obstacles to Creativity." In *A Source Book for Creative Thinking* (Eds.), Sidney J. Parnes and Harold Harding. New York: Charles Scribner's Sons, pp. 106-113.

Wallas, Graham. *The Art of Thought*. London: Jonathan Cape, 1926.

Watson, Kenneth W. "Efficiency Versus Process." *Public Welfare*, Summer, 1983, pp. 19-23.

Whitfield, P. R. *Creativity in Industry*. Middlesex, England: Penguin Books, 1975.

Wilford, John Noble. "Nobel Winner is Loner in the Laboratory." *Globe and Mail*. October 13, 1983.

York, Reginald O. *Human Service Planning: Concepts, Tools and Methods*. Chapel Hill: The University of North Carolina Press, 1982.

Index